BLUE SWAN COSMIC BATH & BODY

BLUE SWAN COSMIC BATH & BODY

Disclaimer for Recipes, Rituals, and Elixirs
The recipes and rituals shared in this book are intended for educational and inspirational purposes only. Results may vary depending on your skin type, personal sensitivities, and environmental factors. Please do a patch test before using any product on your skin. These elixirs and rituals are not intended to diagnose, treat, or cure any medical condition. Always consult with a healthcare provider before making significant changes to your wellness routine.

BLUE SWAN COSMIC BATH & BODY

Introduction

Welcome, my fellow goddesses, to the ultimate guide to indulgence, empowerment, and total transformation! You're not here to take a basic bath; you're about to immerse yourself in a divine ritual that celebrates your strength, beauty, and boundless energy.

This isn't your run-of-the-mill self-care book—oh no, darling—this is a journey into the cosmic realms where ancient elixirs meet modern magic. Whether you're prepping for the biggest event of your life or just need to recharge from life's constant hustle, I've got you covered. So light those candles, set the vibe, and get ready to soak in the essence of luxury. Your transformation starts here!

BLUE SWAN COSMIC BATH & BODY

Dedication

To my Divine Father, God—my ultimate guide, protector, and best friend. This book is a tribute to the love that transcends time and space. You have shaped my world, and your light is the source of all my joy, healing, and purpose. I love You more than I love myself, and that is saying something. May this book reflect even a fraction of the endless love, grace, and beauty that You've shown me.

Thank You for guiding my hands and heart in everything I create.

BLUE SWAN COSMIC BATH & BODY

Copyright Disclaimer Page

BLUE SWAN COSMIC BATH & BODY

Author's Page

Hello, beautiful souls! I'm S. Petit, and I'm beyond excited to share my journey of cosmic wellness, luxurious rituals, and healing elixirs with you. This book is the culmination of years spent blending ancient practices with modern self-care techniques, all with the goal of empowering you to embrace your divine essence. Whether it's a bath that makes you feel like royalty or a potion that heals your soul, my mission is to help you indulge in the sacred art of self-love. Reach out to me anytime at 4onlyshay@gmail.com—I'd love to hear your stories and connect on this magical journey.

BLUE SWAN COSMIC BATH & BODY

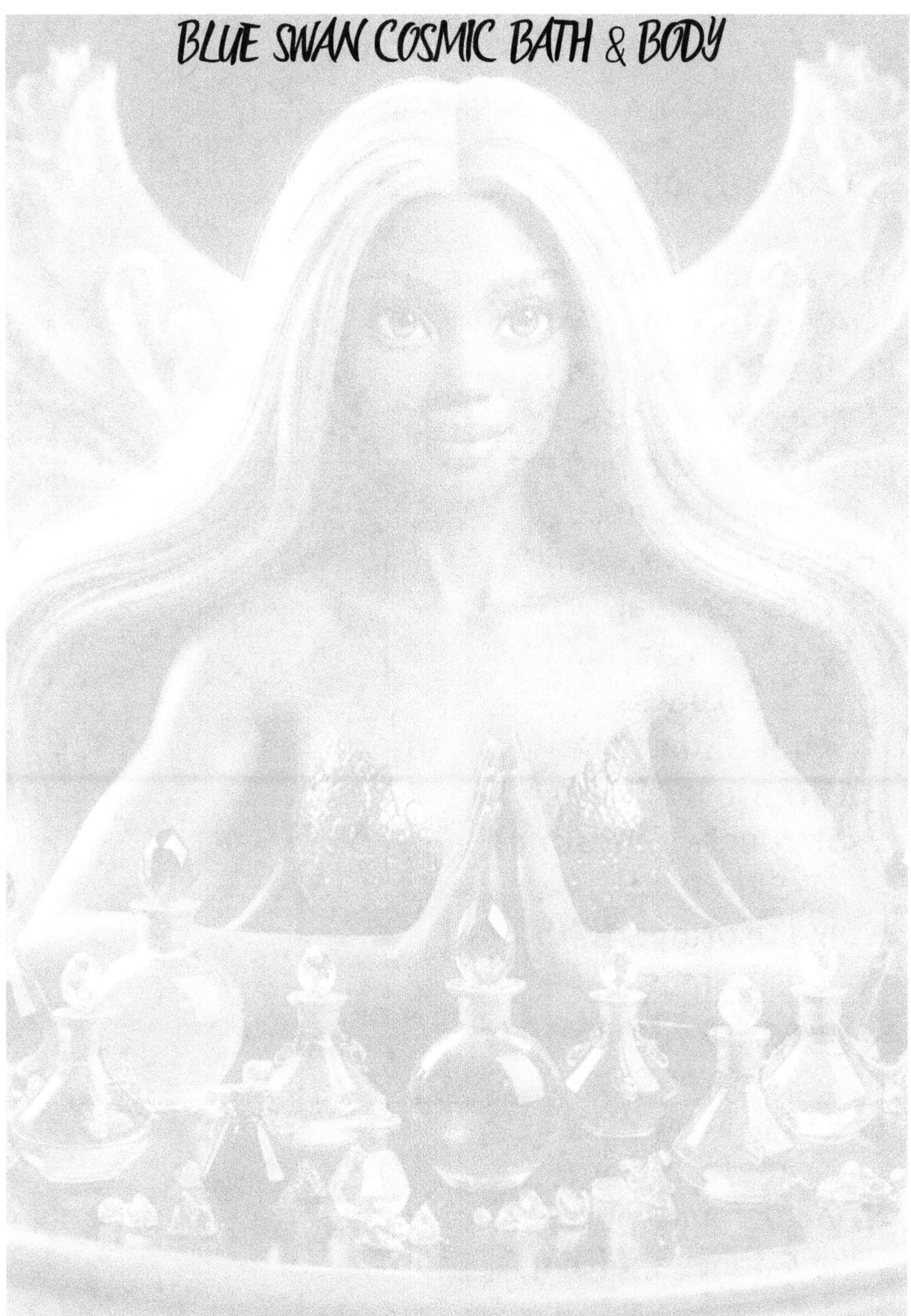

BLUE SWAN COSMIC BATH & BODY

Table of Contents

BLUE SWAN COSMIC BATH & BODY

Elevate Your Skin & Spirit with Cosmic Care

Weave a rich, evocative story around your brand and products:

Divine Inspiration: Share the spiritual and cosmic inspiration behind your brand, linking your products to ancient beauty rituals or divine energy.

Rare Ingredient Stories: Highlight the origins of rare ingredients like saffron, oud, or gemstones, and how they've been used for centuries by royalty or in sacred rituals.

Customer Journeys: Showcase testimonials or customer stories, focusing on how the products made them feel pampered, rejuvenated, and connected to something greater.

BLUE SWAN COSMIC BATH & BODY

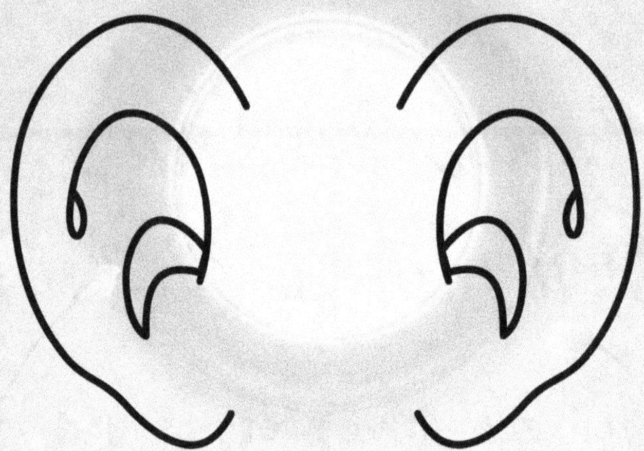

Protecting your ears and maintaining pH balance while taking a bath is important for overall comfort and health.
Here are some tips to help you achieve that:

By taking these steps, you can protect your ears and maintain a healthy pH balance during your bath.
This will help ensure a more enjoyable and comfortable bathing experience while promoting overall skin health.

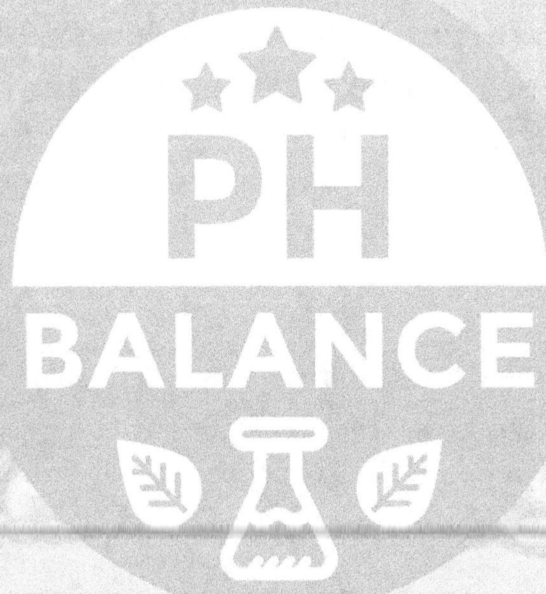

BLUE SWAN COSMIC BATH & BODY

Protecting Your Ears

Use Earplugs:
Invest in waterproof earplugs designed for bathing. These can help keep water out of your ears and prevent discomfort or infections.

Avoid Submerging Your Head:
If you prefer to keep your hair dry, avoid submerging your head underwater. You can also lean back and keep your ears above the waterline.

Swim Cap:
A swim cap can provide a barrier to keep water out of your ears while allowing you to enjoy your bath.

Tilt Your Head:
If water does enter your ears, tilt your head to the side to help drain the water out. You can also pull on your earlobe gently while tilting your head.

Dry Your Ears Afterward:
After bathing, gently dry your ears with a towel. You can also use a hairdryer on the lowest setting, held at a distance, to help evaporate any remaining moisture.

BLUE SWAN COSMIC BATH & BODY

Maintaining pH Balance

Choose pH-Balanced Bath Products:
Use bath products (like bath oils, salts, or bubbles) that are pH-balanced. Look for those labeled as such to avoid disrupting your skin's natural pH.

Avoid Harsh Soaps:
Stay away from harsh soaps and cleansers that can strip your skin of its natural oils and upset the pH balance. Opt for gentle, moisturizing cleansers instead.

Add Baking Soda:
Adding a small amount of baking soda (about 1/4 to 1/2 cup) to your bath can help neutralize acidity and maintain a balanced pH level in the water.

Use Vinegar:
Adding a cup of apple cider vinegar to your bath can help balance pH. It may also provide soothing benefits for the skin.

Monitor Water Temperature:
Avoid using excessively hot water, which can strip oils from your skin and upset the pH balance. Opt for warm (not hot) water instead.

Stay Hydrated:
Drinking plenty of water before and after your bath helps maintain hydration and can support your skin's health and pH balance.

Post-Bath Moisturizing:
After bathing, apply a gentle moisturizer to help lock in moisture and maintain your skin's natural pH balance.

Consult a Dermatologist:
If you frequently experience skin issues or pH imbalance, consider consulting a dermatologist for personalized advice and recommendations.

BLUE SWAN COSMIC BATH & BODY

Here's a simple and organic candle-making recipe that you can try at home!

This recipe uses natural ingredients and essential oils for a soothing and fragrant experience.

BLUE SWAN COSMIC BATH & BODY

Organic Soy Candle Recipe
Ingredients:

Soy wax flakes: 1 pound
(approximately 16 ounces)

Essential oils:

1-2 ounces (your choice, e.g.,
lavender, eucalyptus, or citrus)

Candle wicks: 2
(pre-tabbed, suitable for the size of your container)

Containers: 2 (glass jars or metal tins)

Double boiler:

For melting the wax

Thermometer:

To check wax temperature

Stirring stick:
A wooden spoon or stick for stirring

Pouring pitcher:
For easy pouring of melted wax
Coloring (optional): Natural candle dye or crayon pieces
(if you want colored candles)

BLUE SWAN COSMIC BATH & BODY

Organic Soy Candle Recipe

Here's a simple and organic candle-making recipe that you can try at home!

This recipe uses natural ingredients and essential oils for a soothing and fragrant experience.

Making organic candles is a fun and rewarding project that allows you to customize scents and colors according to your preferences.

Enjoy your beautiful creations in your bathing space or gift them to friends and family!

BLUE SWAN COSMIC BATH & BODY

Organic Soy Candle Recipe

Instructions:

Prepare Your Workspace:

Cover your work surface with newspaper or an old cloth to catch any spills. Make sure your containers are clean and dry.

Measure the Wax:

Measure out 1 pound of soy wax flakes. This will make about 16 ounces of finished candles.

Melt the Wax:

Fill the bottom pot of your double boiler with water and place it on the stove over medium heat.
Add the soy wax flakes to the top pot and let them melt, stirring occasionally until fully liquefied. Use the thermometer to check the temperature; the ideal melting point is around 170-180°F (77-82°C).

Add Color (Optional):

If you want to color your candle, add natural candle dye or a small piece of crayon to the melted wax and stir until fully dissolved.

Add Essential Oils:

Once the wax is melted, remove it from heat and let it cool slightly to around 160°F (71°C).
Add your chosen essential oils (1-2 ounces) and stir well to combine. The amount depends on your scent preference; for a stronger scent, use more oil.

BLUE SWAN COSMIC BATH & BODY

Organic Soy Candle Recipe

Prepare the Wicks:

While the wax cools, attach the wick to the center of the container. You can do this by dipping the metal base of the wick into the melted wax, then pressing it down firmly in the center of the container.

Pour the Wax:

Once the wax is at the right temperature, carefully pour it into the prepared containers. Leave a small amount of wax in the pot for topping off the candles later if needed.

Secure the wick in place by using a wick holder or by wrapping the top of the wick around a pencil or chopstick laid across the top of the container.

Let it Set:

Allow the candles to cool at room temperature for a few hours until fully hardened.

Top Off (Optional):

If the surface of your candles has any sinkholes or imperfections, reheat the reserved wax and pour it on top to create a smooth finish.

Trim the Wicks:

Once the candles are fully set, trim the wicks to about 1/4 inch above the surface of the wax.

Cure Your Candles:

For the best scent throw, allow your candles to cure for at least 24 hours before lighting them.

Enjoy:

Light your organic candles and enjoy the soothing scents and ambiance!

BLUE SWAN COSMIC BATH & BODY

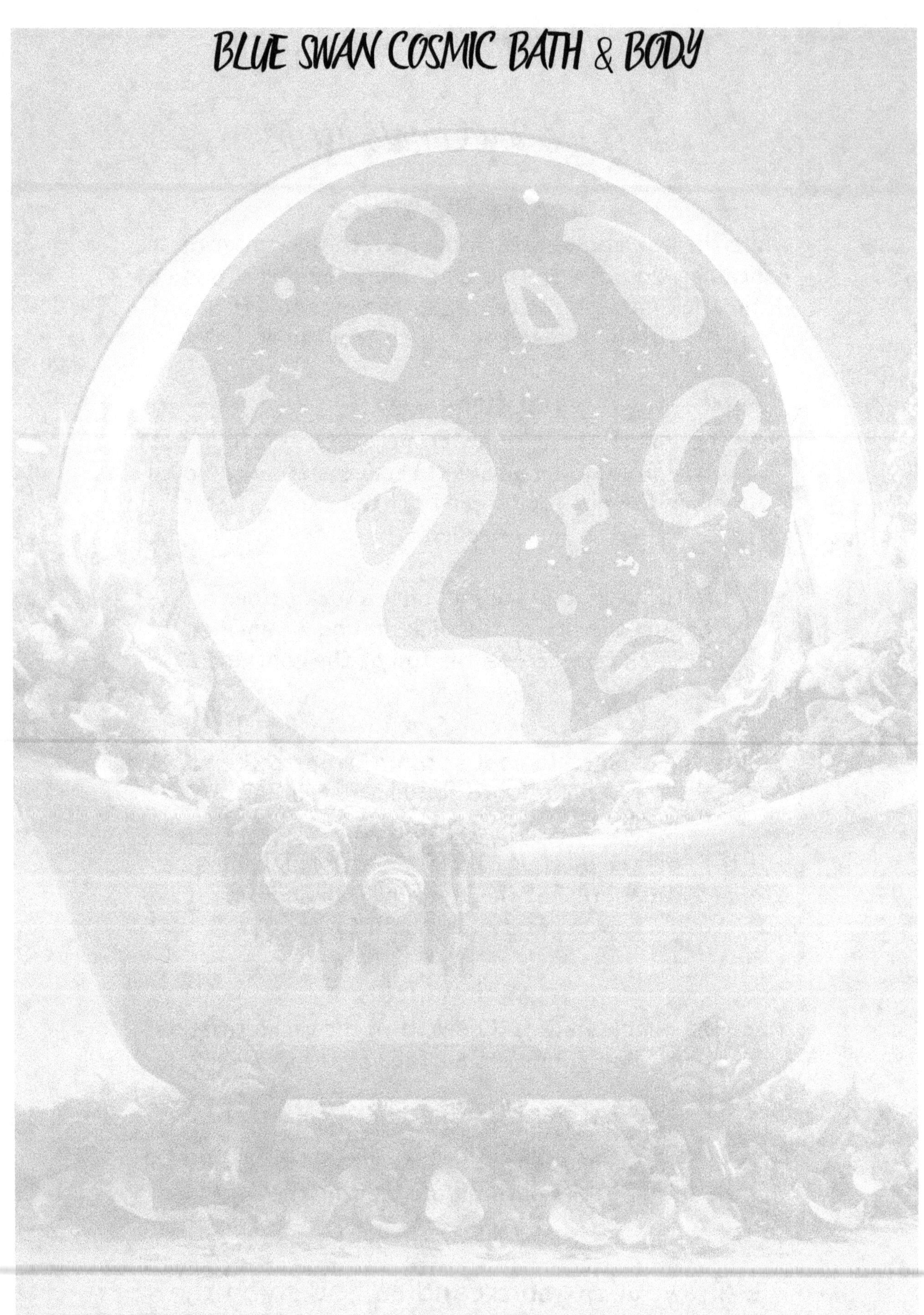

BLUE SWAN COSMIC BATH & BODY

How to Pray in the Bath

Set the Mood:
Begin by preparing your bath. Use warm water, bath salts, or essential oils that resonate with you. Dim the lights or use candles for a soft glow.

Choose Your Intention:
Decide on the intention of your prayer. This could be gratitude, healing, guidance, or simply a moment of peace.

Get Comfortable:
Find a comfortable position in the bath. You might want to sit upright or lean back against the tub, allowing yourself to relax completely.

Begin with Gratitude:
Start your prayer by expressing gratitude for the moment, your body, and the water surrounding you. Acknowledge any blessings in your life.

Use Affirmations or Mantras:
You can repeat affirmations or mantras that resonate with you. This could be something like "I am loved," "I am at peace," or any other phrase that feels right.

Speak from the Heart:
Allow your thoughts and feelings to flow. Speak openly about your desires, hopes, or any burdens you're carrying. Be sincere and authentic in your words.

Visualize:
As you pray, visualize light or energy surrounding you, enveloping you in warmth and comfort. This can enhance your connection to the divine or your higher self.

Listen and Reflect:
After you've spoken your prayer, take a moment to listen. You may not hear a voice, but pay attention to your thoughts and feelings. This is a time for reflection.

Close with Affirmation:
End your prayer with a positive affirmation or a simple "Amen" or "So be it." Thank the universe or your higher power for the experience and any guidance you've received.

Enjoy the Bath:
Allow yourself to relax fully in the bath afterward. Take time to breathe deeply and enjoy the soothing sensations of the water.

BLUE SWAN COSMIC BATH & BODY

Candles That Work Best for Bath Prayers

Scented Candles:
Choose candles with calming scents like lavender, chamomile, or sandalwood. These fragrances can promote relaxation and enhance your spiritual practice.

Meditation Candles:
Look for candles specifically labeled for meditation or spiritual practices. They often come in scents designed to elevate your mood and enhance focus.

Color Symbolism:
White Candles: Represent purity and peace, making them ideal for a calming environment.
Blue Candles: Promote tranquility and spiritual connection.

Green Candles:
Associated with healing and abundance.
Pink Candles: Symbolize love and compassion, perfect for prayers focused on relationships and self-love.

Natural Candles:
Consider beeswax or soy candles, which are more natural alternatives to paraffin candles. They burn cleaner and can enhance the purity of your prayer space.

Crystal-Infused Candles:
Some candles are infused with crystals like rose quartz, amethyst, or clear quartz. These can add an extra layer of energy and intention to your prayers.

Floating Candles:
For a unique touch, use floating candles in your bath. They create a magical ambiance and add a gentle glow to the water.

BLUE SWAN COSMIC BATH & BODY

Praying in the bath can be a transformative experience, allowing you to connect with your spirituality while nurturing your body and mind.

By setting the right ambiance with candles that resonate with your intentions, you can create a sacred space that promotes relaxation, reflection, and renewal.

Enjoy the serenity of the moment as you blend self-care with your spiritual journey!

BLUE SWAN COSMIC BATH & BODY

Bathing has always been about more than just physical cleanliness—it's an act of self-care, spiritual purification, healing, and social connection.

From the elaborate public baths of Rome to the sacred rituals of ancient India and the relaxing hot springs of Japan, bathing continues to evolve as an important part of human culture, reflecting our ongoing relationship with water as a source of life and renewal.

BLUE SWAN COSMIC BATH & BODY

The history of bathing spans thousands of years and is deeply connected to health, spirituality, and social customs across various cultures.

Bathing has evolved from a basic necessity of cleanliness to a significant ritual in many societies, symbolizing purification, healing, and relaxation.

Here's an exploration of how bathing practices developed throughout history:

BLUE SWAN COSMIC BATH & BODY

Ancient Civilizations and Early Bathing Practices

Mesopotamia (3000 BCE)

Bathing has roots in the ancient civilizations of Mesopotamia, where clay tablets mention the use of oils and water for cleanliness and religious purposes. Bathing was both a practical and spiritual act, with temples often including baths for ritual purification.

Egypt (2500 BCE)

The ancient Egyptians were among the first to value bathing as a daily practice, associating cleanliness with religious purity. Wealthy Egyptians would bathe multiple times a day, using scented oils and perfumes. The iconic Queen Cleopatra is said to have bathed in milk to maintain her beauty and youthfulness. Public baths also existed, and bathing was an important social and religious act.

BLUE SWAN COSMIC BATH & BODY

Ancient Greece and Rome

Greece (1000 BCE - 300 BCE)

The Greeks saw bathing as part of their physical health regimen, emphasizing balance between the body and mind. They bathed in natural springs and rivers, often using olive oil as a cleanser. Bathing was connected to gymnasiums where athletes would cleanse themselves after training. Baths were also used to honor the gods, with temples sometimes housing baths for ritual purification.

Rome (500 BCE - 500 CE)

The Romans elevated the art of bathing to an essential part of daily life, with elaborate public baths, or thermae, becoming common by 200 BCE. Roman baths were not just for hygiene but were social centers where people would relax, converse, and conduct business. The Romans heated water using an advanced hypocaust system, and these bathhouses included steam rooms, cold plunges, and massage facilities. Bathing was considered a communal activity for people of all classes, though separate hours or facilities existed for men and women.

BLUE SWAN COSMIC BATH & BODY

Medieval and Renaissance Europe
Medieval Europe (500 CE - 1500 CE)

After the fall of the Roman Empire, the importance of bathing diminished in Europe, partly due to the association of public baths with disease during plagues and epidemics. Christian asceticism also played a role, with the belief that physical cleanliness could lead to spiritual corruption. Bathing became more private, and public baths were less common, especially in Western Europe.

However, in Eastern Europe and the Islamic world, public baths, or hammams, flourished. These were luxurious spaces where both physical and spiritual cleansing occurred.

Renaissance (14th - 17th Century)

With the Renaissance came a revival of bathing traditions, as well as a renewed interest in hygiene and the human body. Wealthier individuals began to enjoy private baths, often scented with herbs and flowers. The invention of plumbing systems and bathing tubs allowed for more elaborate bathing rituals at home, although public baths were still in decline.

Bathing in Asia
India (2000 BCE)

In ancient India, bathing was a sacred practice, integral to Hindu and Ayurvedic traditions. The Indus Valley civilization had advanced drainage systems, and baths were considered essential for spiritual and physical well-being. Ritual purification before prayer and temple visits remains common in Hindu culture, often performed in holy rivers such as the Ganges.

BLUE SWAN COSMIC BATH & BODY

Japan (700 CE - Present)

In Japan, communal bathing has a rich history, with onsen (hot springs) and sento (public bathhouses) being integral to Japanese culture. Onsen, in particular, is revered for its healing properties, due to the mineral content of the spring waters. The Japanese ritual of bathing focuses on relaxation, cleanliness, and rejuvenation, with a strong emphasis on mindfulness and respect for nature.

China (3000 BCE - Present)

In China, bathing was associated with both hygiene and medicinal practices. Herbs and medicinal plants were often used in baths to promote health and treat ailments. Bathing also had a spiritual element, with many religious traditions incorporating water purification rituals.

The Ottoman Empire
And Islamic World
(800 CE - 1900 CE)

Bathing in the Islamic world reached a new level of sophistication, with the hammam becoming a key feature of cities.

Public baths were deeply tied to religious practices, as Muslims are required to cleanse themselves before prayer.

Hammams were also social hubs where people gathered for relaxation and conversation, much like the Roman baths.

They featured steam rooms, cold plunge pools, and massage areas.

.

BLUE SWAN COSMIC BATH & BODY

The Victorian Era (19th Century)
In the 19th century, advancements in plumbing and sanitation in Europe and America transformed bathing into a more private, hygienic activity. The Victorian obsession with cleanliness led to the introduction of bathtubs in homes, though bathing was often still a luxury for the wealthy. Soap became a mass-produced commodity, and medicinal baths gained popularity as a treatment for skin conditions and other ailments.

Modern Bathing (20th Century - Present)
In the 20th century, bathing evolved into a daily routine, aided by widespread access to clean water and indoor plumbing. The luxury spa industry also developed, offering therapeutic baths such as mud baths, mineral baths, and aromatherapy baths for relaxation and healing.

Today, bathing is seen not only as a form of hygiene but also as a way to promote mental well-being, reduce stress, and engage in self-care rituals. Special types of baths, such as salt baths, milk baths, and herbal baths, are popular for their aesthetic and health benefits. The incorporation of essential oils, crystals, and meditation in baths reflects the continuing spiritual connection to water and cleansing.

BLUE SWAN COSMIC BATH & BODY

Cultural and Symbolic Meanings
Across cultures, bathing has been more than just a
means of cleanliness:

Religious Purification:
In Christianity, Judaism, Hinduism, Islam, and other
faiths, bathing or water cleansing rituals have been
used to symbolize spiritual purity and rebirth.

Healing and Detoxification:
Since ancient times, people have believed in the
healing power of water, whether through hot springs,
mineral baths, or herbal infusions.

Social and Communal Gatherings:
Many cultures, from Roman baths to Japanese
onsens, have turned bathing into a social practice
where people relax and bond.

BLUE SWAN COSMIC BATH & BODY

Healing and detoxification through bathing has been a time-honored practice across many cultures, combining the soothing and restorative qualities of water with natural ingredients, minerals, and herbs to cleanse both body and spirit.

The idea behind healing and detoxification baths is to draw out toxins, rejuvenate the skin, ease stress, and promote overall well-being.

Let's explore how baths have historically been used for these purposes and some of the modern-day interpretations of these ancient practices.

BLUE SWAN COSMIC BATH & BODY

Ancient Healing Baths

Throughout history, people have recognized the healing power of water. Ancient civilizations believed in the restorative effects of natural springs and crafted special bathing rituals for health, relaxation, and spiritual cleansing.

Egyptians:

Queen Cleopatra famously bathed in milk to soften her skin and retain a youthful glow. They also used oils, herbs, and salts to heal and beautify the body.

Romans: The Romans built expansive public baths (thermae) centered on healing and socializing. They used mineral-rich hot springs for their anti-inflammatory properties, soaking in warm water to improve circulation, relieve muscle tension, and detoxify.

Japanese Onsen:

In Japan, hot springs, or onsen, are prized for their naturally occurring minerals, such as sulfur, magnesium, and calcium. These baths are believed to heal skin conditions, improve blood flow, and detoxify the body.

Ayurvedic Medicine:

In India, baths infused with herbs like neem or tulsi have long been used to detoxify and heal the body, following the Ayurvedic principles of balancing the body's energies (doshas) and eliminating impurities.

BLUE SWAN COSMIC BATH & BODY

Modern Healing and Detox Baths

Today, many bathing rituals focus on healing through detoxification, using ingredients that promote wellness, relaxation, and purification.

Epsom Salt Baths

One of the most common detox baths, Epsom salt is rich in magnesium sulfate, which is absorbed through the skin during bathing. This process helps relieve muscle aches, reduces inflammation, and flushes toxins from the body. Epsom salt baths are excellent for alleviating stress, improving circulation, and supporting overall detoxification.

Clay Baths

Clay baths, particularly using bentonite clay, are popular for their ability to draw toxins out of the body. Bentonite clay has negatively charged ions, which bind to positively charged toxins and heavy metals, helping to cleanse the skin and body from impurities. Clay baths can also reduce inflammation and soothe irritated skin.

Herbal Detox Baths

Herbs such as lavender, chamomile, rosemary, and eucalyptus are commonly used in healing baths for their therapeutic properties. These herbs can be steeped in hot water and added to the bath or used in essential oil form. They help calm the mind, relieve tension, and promote skin healing.

Apple Cider Vinegar Baths

Apple cider vinegar is known for its antibacterial and antifungal properties. Adding it to a bath helps restore the skin's natural pH balance, cleanse impurities, and soothe skin irritations like eczema or sunburn. It can also help the body detox by drawing out harmful substances.

BLUE SWAN COSMIC BATH & BODY

Spiritual Cleansing and Healing

Healing baths often extend beyond physical benefits, providing emotional and spiritual purification.

Full Moon Baths:

A full moon bath is a spiritual detoxification ritual where participants soak in mineral-rich water under the full moon's light, often adding herbs, oils, or crystals to enhance the spiritual experience. The full moon is believed to amplify the detoxification process, helping to release emotional burdens and bring clarity.

Crystal Baths:

Incorporating crystals like rose quartz, amethyst, or clear quartz into a bath is said to amplify healing energies. Crystals are thought to realign energy and clear blockages, while the water aids in the absorption of their positive frequencies.

Sound and Aromatherapy: Using essential oils like frankincense and sandalwood or adding singing bowls and soft music can transform a bath into a healing experience. The vibrations from sound healing, combined with aromatherapy, encourage emotional release, clarity, and balance.

BLUE SWAN COSMIC BATH & BODY

How Detox Baths Work
Detox baths work through a process of osmotic pressure, where the body absorbs beneficial minerals through the skin and releases toxins into the bathwater. Warm water opens pores, enabling the skin to sweat out impurities while soaking in nutrients. The minerals and herbs added to the bath further support the body's natural detoxification systems.

Key Benefits:
Toxin Elimination: Detox baths help rid the body of harmful substances, including heavy metals, environmental pollutants, and waste products.
Skin Rejuvenation: Many ingredients in detox baths, such as salts, clays, and oils, have properties that soothe, hydrate, and rejuvenate the skin, making it appear healthier and more radiant.

Stress Relief:
Detox baths help relax the mind and body, reducing stress hormones, calming the nervous system, and promoting better sleep.
Improved Circulation: Soaking in warm water improves circulation, which supports the body's natural detox pathways, including the lymphatic system and blood vessels.

BLUE SWAN COSMIC BATH & BODY

Detox Bath Recipe Example

Here's a simple yet powerful detox bath recipe that
can be customized to your needs:
Healing and Detoxification Bath Recipe
Ingredients:
1 cup Epsom salt
1/2 cup bentonite clay
1/2 cup baking soda
10 drops lavender essential oil (for relaxation)
5 drops eucalyptus essential oil (for detoxification)
1/4 cup apple cider vinegar

Optional:

Rose quartz or amethyst crystal

Instructions:

Fill your bathtub with warm (not too hot) water.
Add the Epsom salt, bentonite clay, and baking soda,
stirring them into the water until they dissolve.
Add the essential oils and apple cider vinegar.
Place your crystal in the bath, if desired, and allow it
to infuse the water with healing energy.

Soak for 20-30 minutes, allowing your body to sweat
and detoxify.
After your bath, rinse off with a cool shower to close
your pores.

Post-Bath Tip:

Hydrate well after a detox bath, as the process can
be dehydrating. Sip water with lemon to further
cleanse the body.

BLUE SWAN COSMIC BATH & BODY

Healing and detox baths serve as powerful rituals for physical, emotional, and spiritual cleansing.

By utilizing ancient practices alongside modern ingredients, these baths can support wellness, rejuvenate the skin, and promote inner balance.

Whether you're looking to heal your body, detox from stress, or deepen your spiritual connection, these baths offer a holistic approach to self-care.

Full moon rituals, including baths, often use specific herbs to enhance spiritual connection, purification, and manifestation.

The full moon is a time of heightened energy, making it ideal for using herbs that align with its themes of reflection, release, and renewal.

Here are some of the best herbs to incorporate into full moon rituals, especially for baths, teas, or incense:

BLUE SWAN COSMIC BATH & BODY

Mugwort (Artemisia vulgaris)
Properties: Psychic awareness, clarity, dream work
Why It's Great: Mugwort is traditionally associated with enhancing intuition and spiritual insight. It's often used during full moon rituals to open the mind and promote lucid dreaming and visions.

How to Use:
Add mugwort to your bath, burn it as incense, or steep it into a tea for meditation or dreamwork.

Lavender (Lavandula)
Properties:
Relaxation, emotional balance, purification
Why It's Great: Lavender is excellent for calming the mind and body, making it perfect for a full moon bath where emotional release and self-care are needed. Its gentle aroma helps create a soothing environment for meditation and relaxation.

How to Use:
Add dried lavender buds to your bath, use lavender essential oil, or drink lavender tea to relax during a full moon ritual.

BLUE SWAN COSMIC BATH & BODY

Rose (Rosa spp.)
Properties: Love, beauty, emotional healing
Why It's Great: Roses are linked to love, beauty, and emotional healing, aligning with the full moon's power of bringing heightened emotions to the surface. Roses can be used to release emotional blockages and open the heart.

How to Use:
Add rose petals to your bath for a luxurious and heart-opening experience or burn rose incense during a full moon ritual for love and healing energy.

Sage (Salvia spp.)
Properties: Cleansing, protection, purification
Why It's Great: Sage is one of the most powerful herbs for cleansing and clearing negative energy, which is especially important during full moon rituals where you may be releasing unwanted emotions, habits, or energies.

How to Use:
Burn sage as part of a smudging ritual to cleanse your space or add sage to your bath to purify and protect your energy field.

BLUE SWAN COSMIC BATH & BODY

Chamomile (Matricaria chamomilla)
Properties:
Calm, peace, healing
Why It's Great:
Chamomile is known for its soothing and calming properties, helping to bring emotional balance during the intensity of a full moon. It can help you release tension and invite peace into your life.
How to Use:
Add chamomile to your bath for relaxation or drink chamomile tea to unwind during full moon reflection.

Yarrow (Achillea millefolium)
Properties:
Protection, courage, psychic opening
Why It's Great:
Yarrow has a long history of use in protection rituals and for psychic development. It helps create energetic boundaries and promotes inner strength, making it a good herb for full moon rituals focused on personal growth and clarity.
How to Use:
Add yarrow to your bath or burn it as incense during full moon ceremonies.

Jasmine (Jasminum officinale)
Properties:
Feminine energy, love, divination
Why It's Great:
Jasmine is strongly connected to lunar energy and is often used for love, divination, and invoking feminine power. Its intoxicating scent encourages relaxation and spiritual insight.
How to Use:
Use jasmine flowers or essential oil in a full moon bath to connect with the moon's energy and enhance your intuition.

BLUE SWAN COSMIC BATH & BODY

Peppermint (Mentha piperita)
Properties:
Mental clarity, purification, renewal
Why It's Great:
Peppermint has refreshing and purifying properties that help cleanse the mind and body. It is particularly useful during a full moon to release mental clutter and invite fresh, new energy.
How to Use:
Add fresh or dried peppermint leaves to your bath to refresh your spirit and promote clarity.

Thyme (Thymus vulgaris)
Properties:
Courage, strength, healing
Why It's Great:
Thyme is an herb of healing and courage, making it ideal for full moon rituals where you seek inner strength and want to release fear or negative energy. It's also used to promote restful sleep and spiritual clarity.
How to Use:
Add thyme to your bath or burn it as incense to invoke courage and healing during the full moon.

Lemon Balm (Melissa officinalis)
Properties:
Emotional balance, healing, calm
Why It's Great:
Lemon balm is a gentle herb known for its ability to soothe anxiety and balance emotions. It's ideal for helping you find peace and emotional release during a full moon.
How to Use:
Add lemon balm leaves to your bath for a calming experience or drink lemon balm tea to reduce stress and connect with your emotions.

BLUE SWAN COSMIC BATH & BODY

Frankincense (Boswellia spp.)
Properties:
Spirituality, purification, protection
Why It's Great:
Frankincense is one of the most sacred herbs, used in spiritual practices to purify the environment and invite higher consciousness. It is excellent for clearing out negative energies during full moon rituals and invoking deep spiritual clarity.
How to Use:
Burn frankincense resin as incense or use frankincense essential oil to enhance the spiritual energy of your full moon bath or meditation.

Dandelion (Taraxacum officinale)
Properties:
Transformation, release, renewal
Why It's Great:
Dandelion is associated with transformation and letting go, which aligns perfectly with the full moon's themes of release and renewal. It's also used to call in abundance and clarity after emotional release.
How to Use:
Add dandelion flowers or leaves to your bath or drink dandelion tea to aid in letting go of negative energy and manifesting new growth.

BLUE SWAN COSMIC BATH & BODY

How to Use Herbs in Full Moon Rituals:
Herbal Baths:
Create an herbal sachet or steep herbs in hot water and add the infusion to your bath. These baths help you absorb the energies of the herbs, cleanse your aura, and align with the full moon's power.

Incense:
Burn dried herbs like sage, lavender, or frankincense to cleanse your space and prepare for full moon rituals. The smoke purifies your surroundings and opens a connection to spiritual realms.

Teas:
Drinking herbal teas made with full moon herbs like chamomile, lavender, or mugwort can promote relaxation, emotional release, and enhance intuitive insights.

Oils and Essential Oils:
You can add essential oils derived from these herbs into your bath or anoint your body with them to deepen your connection to the lunar energy.

By using these herbs during your full moon rituals, you align yourself with ancient traditions and tap into their healing properties, creating a space for reflection, emotional release, and spiritual growth.

BATH HERB TEA BLENDS

Here's a list of bath herb tea blends specifically for skin cleansing and detoxification.

These can be steeped in hot water and added to your bath for a purifying and soothing experience:

BLUE SWAN COSMIC BATH & BODY
BATH HERB TEA BLENDS

Sage & Rosemary Detox Bath
Ingredients:
Sage leaves, rosemary sprigs, and thyme
Benefits:
Sage is cleansing and purifying, rosemary enhances circulation, and thyme has antibacterial properties, making this blend ideal for a deep skin cleanse.
How to Use:
Steep the herbs in boiling water for 20-30 minutes and pour the strained infusion into your bath.

Dandelion & Burdock Root Detox Blend
Ingredients:
Dried dandelion root, burdock root, and nettle leaves
Benefits:
Dandelion and burdock root are powerful detoxifiers, helping to clear impurities from the skin. Nettle soothes and nourishes irritated skin.
How to Use:
Steep the herbs in hot water for 20-25 minutes, strain them and add to your bath for a skin-cleansing detox.

Lemon Balm & Peppermint Refreshing Blend
Ingredients:
Lemon balm leaves, peppermint, and dried lemon peel
Benefits:
Lemon balm helps balance oily skin, peppermint refreshes, and lemon peel provides a mild exfoliation for smooth, clear skin.
How to Use:
Steep the herbs in hot water for 15-20 minutes and pour the tea into your bath.

BLUE SWAN COSMIC BATH & BODY
BATH HERB TEA BLENDS

Lemon Balm & Peppermint Refreshing Blend
Ingredients: Lemon balm leaves, peppermint, and dried lemon peel

Benefits:
Lemon balm helps balance oily skin, peppermint refreshes, and lemon peel provides a mild exfoliation for smooth, clear skin.

How to Use:
Steep the herbs in hot water for 15-20 minutes and pour the tea into your bath.

Milk Thistle & Fennel Seed Detox Bath
Ingredients: Milk thistle seeds, fennel seeds, and chamomile flowers

Benefits:
Milk thistle detoxifies the skin, fennel helps reduce puffiness, and chamomile calms and soothes. This is ideal for detoxifying and firming the skin.

How to Use:
Steep in hot water for 20 minutes, strain, and add the infusion to your bath.

Jasmine & Lemon Verbena Cleansing Bath
Ingredients:
Jasmine flowers, lemon verbena, and mint leaves

Benefits: Jasmine softens and hydrates the skin, while lemon verbena detoxifies and cleanses, leaving the skin refreshed.

How to Use: Steep
the herbs in boiling water for 15 minutes, strain, and pour into the bath.

Basil & Peppermint Skin Clarifying Bath
Ingredients:
Basil leaves, peppermint, and green tea

Benefits:
Basil acts as a skin toner, reducing blemishes and improving clarity. Peppermint refreshes the skin, and green tea provides antioxidant protection.

How to Use:
Steep for 20 minutes, strain, and add the herbal tea to your bath for a refreshing skin cleanse.

BLUE SWAN COSMIC BATH & BODY
BATH HERB TEA BLENDS

Calendula & Chamomile Blend
Ingredients:
Calendula petals, chamomile flowers, and lavender buds
Benefits:
Calendula is known for its skin healing and anti-inflammatory properties, while chamomile soothes irritated skin. Lavender adds a calming, relaxing touch.
How to Use:
Steep the herbs in hot water for 15-20 minutes and pour the infusion into your bath.

Rose & Hibiscus Blend
Ingredients:
Dried rose petals, hibiscus flowers, and lemon peel
Benefits:
Rose petals help maintain the skin's moisture balance and promote a glowing complexion, while hibiscus has natural alpha-hydroxy acids that gently exfoliate and brighten the skin.
How to Use:
Steep for 20 minutes and pour the infusion into a warm bath for a refreshing skin cleanse.

Green Tea & Mint Detox Blend
Ingredients:
Green tea leaves, peppermint, and eucalyptus leaves
Benefits:
Green tea is packed with antioxidants that detoxify and refresh the skin. Mint and eucalyptus provide a cooling, invigorating sensation that helps with skin clarity.
How to Use:
Steep the leaves in hot water, strain, and add the infused tea to your bath.

Lavender & Oatmeal Soothing Bath
Ingredients:
Lavender buds, oatmeal, and chamomile flowers
Benefits:
Lavender soothes irritation, oatmeal relieves dry, itchy skin, and chamomile provides anti-inflammatory effects. This bath is great for sensitive or irritated skin.
How to Use:
Mix the ingredients, steep in hot water for 20 minutes, and add the strained infusion to your bath.

BLUE SWAN COSMIC BATH & BODY

Tips for Enhancing Your Anxiety-Relief Bath:

Set the Mood:
Use soft lighting like candles or dimmed lights. You can also use colored lights (blue for calm, pink for love).
Add Music: Play calming, meditative music or nature sounds.
Breathe Deeply: Practice mindful breathing to further release anxiety.

Aftercare:
Moisturize your skin with a luxurious body oil or cream post-bath for ultimate pampering.

These Blue Swan Cosmic
Bath & Body recipes are designed to offer a calming, anxiety-reducing experience with luxurious ingredients that nourish both your skin and your spirit.

INTOXICATING AND RELAXING BATHS

Here are 10 recipes for intoxicating and relaxing baths that combine aromatic ingredients, essential oils, and soothing elements to create a serene bathing experience:

BLUE SWAN COSMIC BATH & BODY
INTOXICATING AND RELAXING BATHS

Usage Tips:

Preparation:
For maximum effect, add the mixture to your bathwater while it's running to help dissolve the salts and oils.

Ambiance:
Consider lighting candles, playing soft music, and dimming the lights to enhance relaxation during your bath.

Hydration:
Drink water before and after your bath to stay hydrated.

Enjoy your luxurious and intoxicating bathing experiences!

BLUE SWAN COSMIC BATH & BODY
INTOXICATING AND RELAXING BATHS

Lavender Dream Bath
Ingredients:
1 cup Epsom salt
1/2 cup dried lavender flowers
10 drops of lavender essential oil
1 tablespoon carrier oil (like jojoba or sweet almond)
Instructions:
Combine the Epsom salt and dried lavender. Add the essential oil and carrier oil. Mix well and add to warm running water.

Rose Petal Oasis Bath
Ingredients:
1 cup sea salt
1/2 cup dried rose petals
10 drops of rose essential oil
2 tablespoons coconut oil
Instructions:
Blend the sea salt and rose petals. Mix in the essential oil and melted coconut oil. Add to the bathwater for a romantic soak.

Citrus Bliss Bath
Ingredients:
1 cup baking soda
1/2 cup sea salt
Zest of 1 lemon and 1 orange
10 drops sweet orange essential oil
5 drops lemon essential oil
Instructions:
Combine all ingredients in a bowl. Add to warm bathwater to invigorate your senses.

BLUE SWAN COSMIC BATH & BODY
INTOXICATING AND RELAXING BATHS

Chamomile Serenity Bath
Ingredients:
1 cup Epsom salt
1/2 cup dried chamomile flowers
10 drops of chamomile essential oil
2 tablespoons honey
Instructions:
Mix the Epsom salt and dried chamomile. Add the essential oil and honey, stirring until combined. Pour into a warm bath.

Minty Fresh Bath
Ingredients:
1 cup sea salt
1/2 cup dried peppermint leaves
10 drops peppermint essential oil
1/4 cup coconut milk
Instructions:
Combine sea salt and peppermint leaves. Add peppermint oil and coconut milk. Mix and pour into warm bathwater for a refreshing experience.

Spiced Cinnamon Bath
Ingredients:
1 cup Epsom salt
1 tablespoon ground cinnamon
10 drops cinnamon essential oil
1/4 cup olive oil
Instructions:
Mix Epsom salt with ground cinnamon. Add the essential oil and olive oil. Stir well and add to the bath for a cozy, warming soak.

BLUE SWAN COSMIC BATH & BODY

INTOXICATING AND RELAXING BATHS

Jasmine & Ylang Ylang Luxurious Bath
Ingredients:
1 cup Himalayan pink salt
1/2 cup dried jasmine flowers
10 drops ylang-ylang essential oil
2 tablespoons sweet almond oil
Instructions:
Combine Himalayan pink salt with jasmine flowers. Add ylang-ylang oil and sweet almond oil. Mix thoroughly and add to the warm water.

Exotic Oud & Vanilla Bath
Ingredients:
1 cup Epsom salt
1/2 cup dried vanilla bean pods or 2 tablespoons vanilla extract
10 drops oud essential oil
1/4 cup carrier oil (like grapeseed oil)
Instructions:
Mix Epsom salt with vanilla and oud oil. Stir in the carrier oil. Add to a warm bath for an exotic and soothing experience.

Coconut & Lime Refreshing Bath
Ingredients:
1 cup sea salt
1/2 cup dried coconut flakes
Zest of 2 limes
10 drops lime essential oil
1/4 cup coconut oil
Instructions:
Combine sea salt, coconut flakes, and lime zest. Add lime essential oil and melted coconut oil. Mix well and pour into warm bathwater.

BLUE SWAN COSMIC BATH & BODY

INTOXICATING AND RELAXING BATHS

Jasmine & Ylang Ylang Luxurious Bath

Ingredients:

1 cup Himalayan pink salt
1/2 cup dried jasmine flowers
10 drops ylang-ylang essential oil
2 tablespoons sweet almond oil

Instructions:

Combine Himalayan pink salt with jasmine flowers. Add ylang-ylang oil and sweet almond oil. Mix thoroughly and add to the warm water.

Exotic Oud & Vanilla Bath

Ingredients:

1 cup Epsom salt
1/2 cup dried vanilla bean pods or 2 tablespoons vanilla extract
10 drops oud essential oil
1/4 cup carrier oil (like grapeseed oil)

Instructions:

Mix Epsom salt with vanilla and oud oil. Stir in the carrier oil. Add to a warm bath for an exotic and soothing experience.

Coconut & Lime Refreshing Bath

Ingredients:

1 cup sea salt
1/2 cup dried coconut flakes
Zest of 2 limes
10 drops lime essential oil
1/4 cup coconut oil

Instructions:

Combine sea salt, coconut flakes, and lime zest. Add lime essential oil and melted coconut oil. Mix well and pour into warm bathwater.

BLUE SWAN COSMIC BATH & BODY

INTOXICATING AND RELAXING BATHS

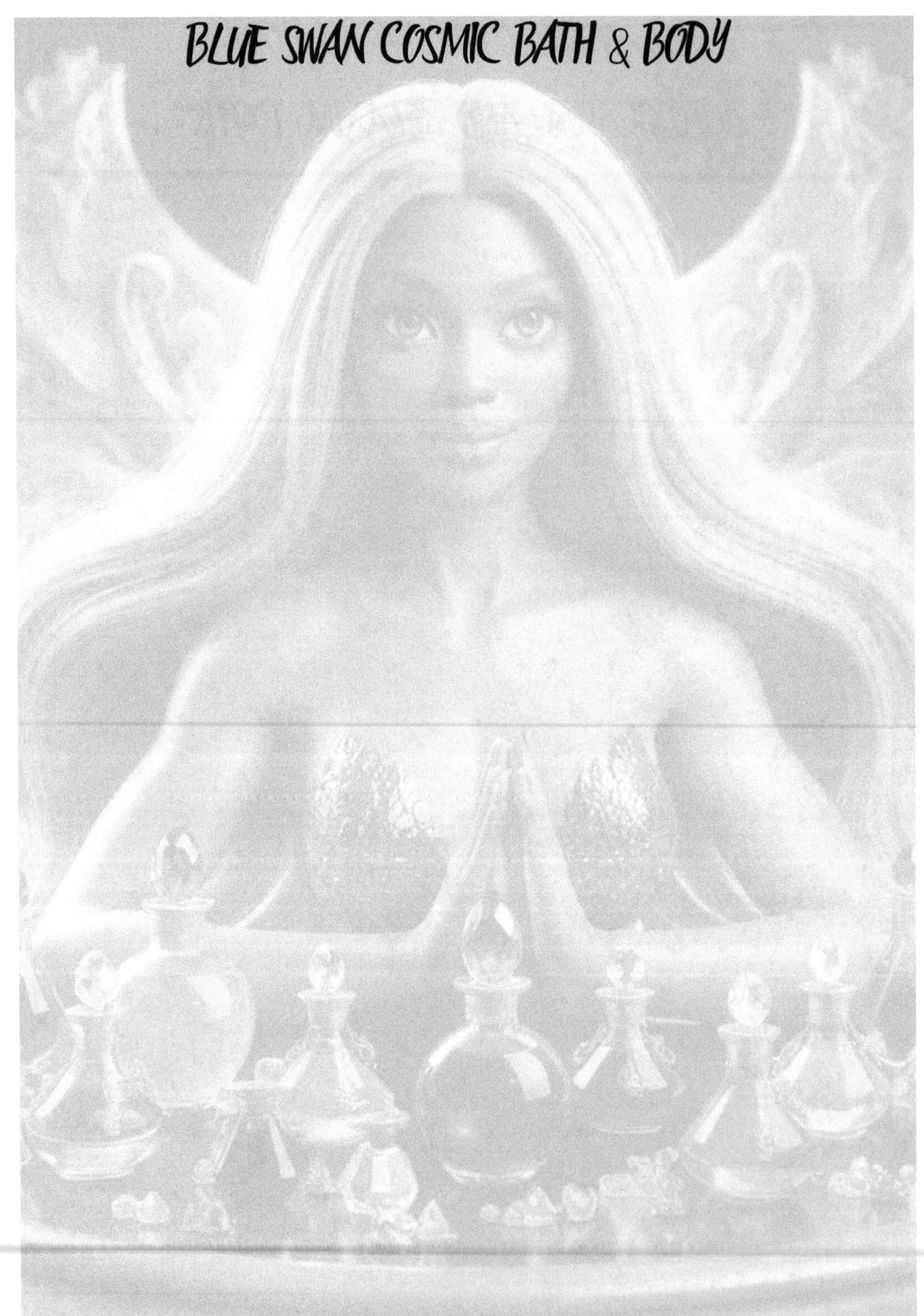

BLUE SWAN COSMIC BATH & BODY

BLUE SWAN COSMIC BATH & BODY

CARRIER OILS

Sweet Almond Oil
Benefits: Moisturizing, rich in vitamins A and E, good for all skin types.
Use: Great for sensitive skin and a popular choice for massage oils.

Jojoba Oil
Benefits: Mimics skin sebum, non-comedogenic, good for all skin types.
Use: Excellent for moisturizing without clogging pores.

Coconut Oil
Benefits: Deeply moisturizing, antibacterial, and antifungal.
Use: Ideal for dry skin and can be used as a makeup remover.

Grapeseed Oil
Benefits: Lightweight, absorbs quickly, rich in antioxidants.
Use: Suitable for oily skin and can help balance oil production.

Argan Oil
Benefits: Rich in vitamin E and fatty acids, excellent for hydration.
Use: Good for dry and aging skin, often used in hair care.

Olive Oil
Benefits: Rich in antioxidants, deeply nourishing.
Use: Great for dry skin, can be used as a massage oil or in hair treatments.

Avocado Oil
Benefits: Highly moisturizing, rich in fatty acids and vitamins.
Use: Ideal for dry or mature skin, enhances elasticity.

Hemp Seed Oil
Benefits: Rich in omega fatty acids, and anti-inflammatory.
Use: Beneficial for acne-prone and sensitive skin.

Rosehip Oil
Benefits: Rich in vitamins A and C, good for skin regeneration.
Use: Helps rduce scars and fine lines.

BLUE SWAN COSMIC BATH & BODY

ESSENTIAL OILS

Lavender Oil
Benefits: Calming, promotes relaxation and sleep.
Use: Perfect for reducing stress and enhancing sleep quality.

Peppermint Oil
Benefits: Refreshing, invigorating, can relieve headaches.
Use: Good for energizing and improving focus.

Tea Tree Oil
Benefits: Antibacterial, antifungal, helps with acne.
Use is Ideal for treating blemishes and skin infections.

Eucalyptus Oil
Benefits: Refreshing, clears respiratory passages.
Use: Good for alleviating cold symptoms and muscle pain.

Frankincense Oil
Benefits: Promotes relaxation, has anti-inflammatory properties.
Use: Helpful for reducing stress and improving skin tone.

Lemon Oil
Benefits: Uplifting, refreshing, antibacterial.
Use: Great for enhancing mood and cleansing properties.

Rose Oil
Benefits: Uplifting, helps with emotional balance, good for skin.
Use Ideal for creating a romantic or calming atmosphere.

Ylang Ylang Oil
Benefits: Balancing, reduces stress, can improve mood.
Use: Good for enhancing relaxation and promoting positive feelings.

Bergamot Oil
Benefits: Uplifting, can help reduce anxiety and stress.
Use: Useful for improving mood and promoting relaxation.

BLUE SWAN COSMIC BATH & BODY

OILS AND ESSENTIAL OILS
BLENDS

Popular Combinations

Relaxing Blend

Carrier: Sweet Almond Oil

Essential Oils: Lavender and Chamomile

Invigorating Blend

Carrier: Grapeseed Oil

Essential Oils: Peppermint and Lemon

Balancing Blend

Carrier: Jojoba Oil

Essential Oils: Ylang Ylang and Bergamot

Skin Nourishing Blend

Carrier: Rosehip Oil

Essential Oils: Frankincense and Tea Tree

Soothing Blend

Carrier: Coconut Oil

Essential Oils: Eucalyptus and Lavender

BLUE SWAN COSMIC BATH & BODY

OILS AND ESSENTIAL OILS

How to Use Carrier and Essential Oils Together
Dilution Ratio:
A common dilution ratio is 2-3% essential oil to carrier oil for topical applications. This typically translates to about 12 drops of essential oil per 1 ounce (30 ml) of carrier oil.
Mixing:
Combine the carrier oil and essential oils in a clean, dark glass bottle to protect the oils from light.
Application:
Apply the blend to the desired areas (e.g., pulse points, affected skin areas) or add it to a warm bath for a relaxing soak.
Patch Test:
Always perform a patch test before applying a new blend to ensure there are no adverse reactions.
This guide should help you explore the benefits of carrier and essential oils for your skincare and wellness routine!

BLUE SWAN COSMIC BATH & BODY
INCENSE

BLUE SWAN COSMIC BATH & BODY

How to Make Incense at Home
(Step-by-Step Guide)

Tips:
You can experiment with different blends and proportions to find your ideal exotic scent.

When using essential oils, always add them gradually to avoid making the mixture too wet.

Store your incense in a cool, dry place to preserve the fragrance.

BLUE SWAN COSMIC BATH & BODY

How to Make Incense at Home
(Step-by-Step Guide)

Gather your materials:
Incense-making requires a few basic tools like a mortar and pestle for grinding, a mixing bowl, essential oils, and natural resins, herbs, or powders.

Choose your base:
Popular bases for incense include agarwood (oud), sandalwood, frankincense, and copal. These are great for grounding and carrying the fragrance of the other ingredients.

Add the aromatics:
Choose exotic herbs, spices, flowers, or essential oils to create your unique scent. Ground these ingredients into a fine powder.

Combine the ingredients:
Slowly blend the powders and resins, adding a few drops of essential oil as needed to create a damp, moldable mixture. Shape the incense: Depending on your preference, you can form the incense into cones, sticks, or small molds. Use your hands to gently shape the mixture.

Dry the incense:
Allow the shaped incense to air dry for at least 2-3 days, ensuring they harden fully before use.

Burn and enjoy:
Once dry, light the incense in a safe, heat-proof dish. Allow the aroma to fill your space with an exotic, luxurious fragrance.

BLUE SWAN COSMIC BATH & BODY

How to Make Incense at Home (Step-by-Step Guide)

The best resins for incense are known for their aromatic qualities, spiritual properties, and ability to burn cleanly. Here's a list of the most popular and effective resins for incense making:

BLUE SWAN COSMIC BATH & BODY

How to Make Incense at Home
(Step-by-Step Guide)

Best for Specific Purposes:
- Spiritual Work & Meditation: Frankincense, Sandalwood, Myrrh
- Protection & Cleansing: Dragon's Blood, Copal, Galbanum
- Relaxation & Mood Elevation: Benzoin, Amber, Myrrh
- Energy & Clarity: Copal, Damar, Frankincense

When making incense, combining these resins with herbs and essential oils can create a more complex and potent blend tailored to your specific needs.

BLUE SWAN COSMIC BATH & BODY
How to Make Incense at Home
(Step-by-Step Guide)

Frankincense
Aroma: Sweet, woody, and slightly citrusy
Properties: Purifying, grounding, and uplifting
Uses: Traditionally used in spiritual rituals, meditation, and relaxation. It helps promote feelings of peace and focus.

Myrrh
Aroma: Warm, earthy, and slightly medicinal
Properties: Grounding, calming, and protective
Uses: Often used for cleansing, meditation, and healing purposes. Myrrh is deeply grounding and can help with emotional balance.

Copal
Aroma: Fresh, sweet, and slightly pine-like
Properties: Cleansing, energizing, and uplifting
Uses: Frequently used in spiritual ceremonies, especially in Central and South American traditions. Copal clears negative energy and elevates the mood.

Dragon's Blood
Aroma: Sweet, spicy, and slightly smoky
Properties: Protective, energizing, and purifying
Uses: Known for its protective and healing properties, Dragon's Blood is often used in rituals for courage, power, and to enhance other incense blends.

Benzoin
Aroma: Sweet, vanilla-like with balsamic undertones
Properties: Soothing, uplifting, and calming
Uses: Benzoin is often used to calm the mind and boost mood. Its sweet scent makes it a great addition to other resins in incense blends.

BLUE SWAN COSMIC BATH & BODY

How to Make Incense at Home
(Step-by-Step Guide)

Amber Resin
Aroma: Warm, sweet, and slightly musky
Properties: Grounding, calming, and balancing
Uses: Often used to promote relaxation and emotional balance. It's also believed to attract positive energy and is commonly used in luxury incense blends.

Sandalwood Resin
Aroma: Soft, woody, and creamy
Properties: Calming, grounding, and purifying
Uses: Sandalwood is revered in spiritual practices for its ability to enhance meditation, promote relaxation, and cleanse spaces.

Opoponax (Sweet Myrrh)
Aroma: Sweet, spicy, and earthy
Properties: Grounding, balancing, and protective
Uses: Often used in protective rituals and to relieve anxiety, Opoponax has a deeply calming and grounding effect.

Damar
Aroma: Light, citrusy, and slightly pine-like
Properties: Uplifting and purifying
Uses: Damar is used to clear the air and bring clarity of mind. It's a good resin to burn for mental focus and fresh energy.

Galbanum
Aroma: Sharp, green, and earthy
Properties: Purifying, protective, and meditative
Uses: Galbanum is often used in incense for spiritual and meditative purposes. It's also associated with protection and healing rituals.

BLUE SWAN COSMIC BATH & BODY

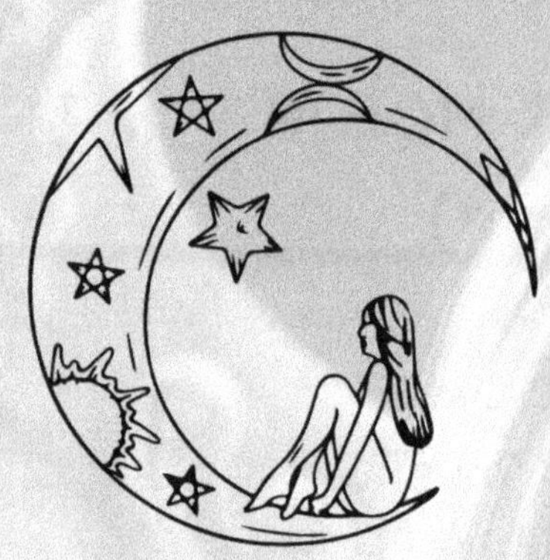

FULL MOON BATH

Using incense during a full moon bath can transform the experience into a deeply spiritual and rejuvenating ritual.

The full moon is a time of heightened energy, completion, and reflection, and incense can amplify these energies in the following ways:

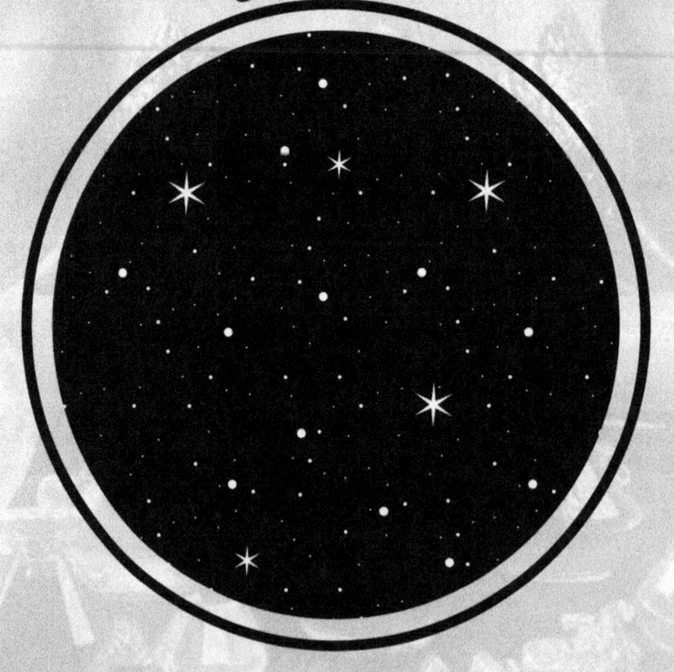

BLUE SWAN COSMIC BATH & BODY

FULL MOON BATH

Purification of the Space

Incense has been used for centuries to cleanse spaces of negative energy. Before your full moon bath, burning incense like frankincense, myrrh, or copal can clear the energy in your bathroom, creating a sacred and serene environment. This helps you enter the bath with a clear mind and a purified space, making your experience more intentional.

Enhanced Meditation and Focus

The full moon is a powerful time for introspection, meditation, and connecting with your inner self. Incense like sandalwood, amber, or lavender can help calm the mind and promote deeper meditation, allowing you to focus on your intentions and manifestations. As the fragrant smoke fills the air, it guides you into a peaceful state, helping you release what no longer serves you and open up to new possibilities.

Aligning with Lunar Energies

Specific resins and herbs burned as incense can align with lunar energies. For instance, jasmine and frankincense resonate with the divine feminine and lunar energy, promoting emotional balance and spiritual clarity. These scents help you sync with the moon's cycles, enhancing the bath's transformational power.

BLUE SWAN COSMIC BATH & BODY

FULL MOON BATH

A full moon bath is often used to release emotional baggage, reflect on past events, and heal. Incense like dragon blood, opoponax, or benzoin is potent for emotional release and protection. Burning these resins can enhance the healing process, encouraging emotional detox and renewal.

Amplifying Manifestations and Intentions

The full moon is an optimal time for manifestation rituals. Burning incense during your bath can help amplify your intentions. For example, using frankincense or copal can create a powerful atmosphere to focus on manifesting goals, while patchouli or cinnamon can be burned to attract abundance, love, or success.

Deepening Relaxation and Detoxification

Full moon baths are often about relaxation and physical detoxification. Incense with soothing properties like lavender, sandalwood, or rose can help relax the mind and body, making the bath a more immersive and restful experience. These scents, combined with the water's detoxifying effects, help you let go of stress and tension.

Creating a Ritual Atmosphere

Using incense during a full moon bath creates a ceremonial feel, turning a simple bath into a sacred ritual. The act of lighting incense, watching the smoke, and feeling the gentle aroma connects you to ancient traditions of honoring the moon. It heightens your awareness of the moment and the cyclical nature of life, making the bath a more profound experience.

BLUE SWAN COSMIC BATH & BODY

FULL MOON BATH

Suggested Incense for Full Moon Baths:
Frankincense: Purification, spiritual clarity
Myrrh: Healing, grounding
Jasmine: Feminine energy, emotional balance
Dragon's Blood: Protection, energy clearing
Lavender: Relaxation, peace
Sandalwood: Meditation, mental focus
By incorporating incense into your full moon bath ritual, you create an elevated experience that connects you with the moon's energy, helps you release and manifest, and brings you closer to a state of inner peace and balance.

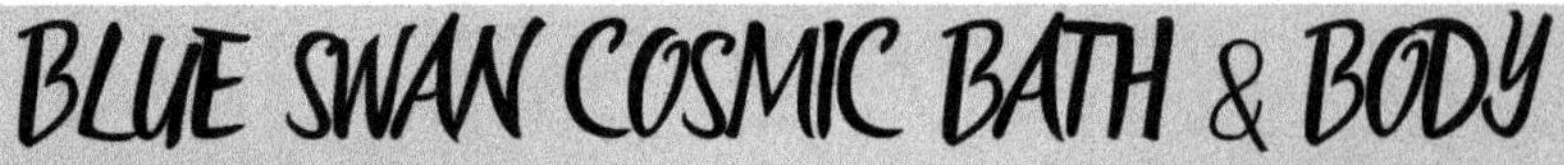

BLUE SWAN COSMIC BATH & BODY

How to Make Incense at Home
(Step-by-Step Guide)

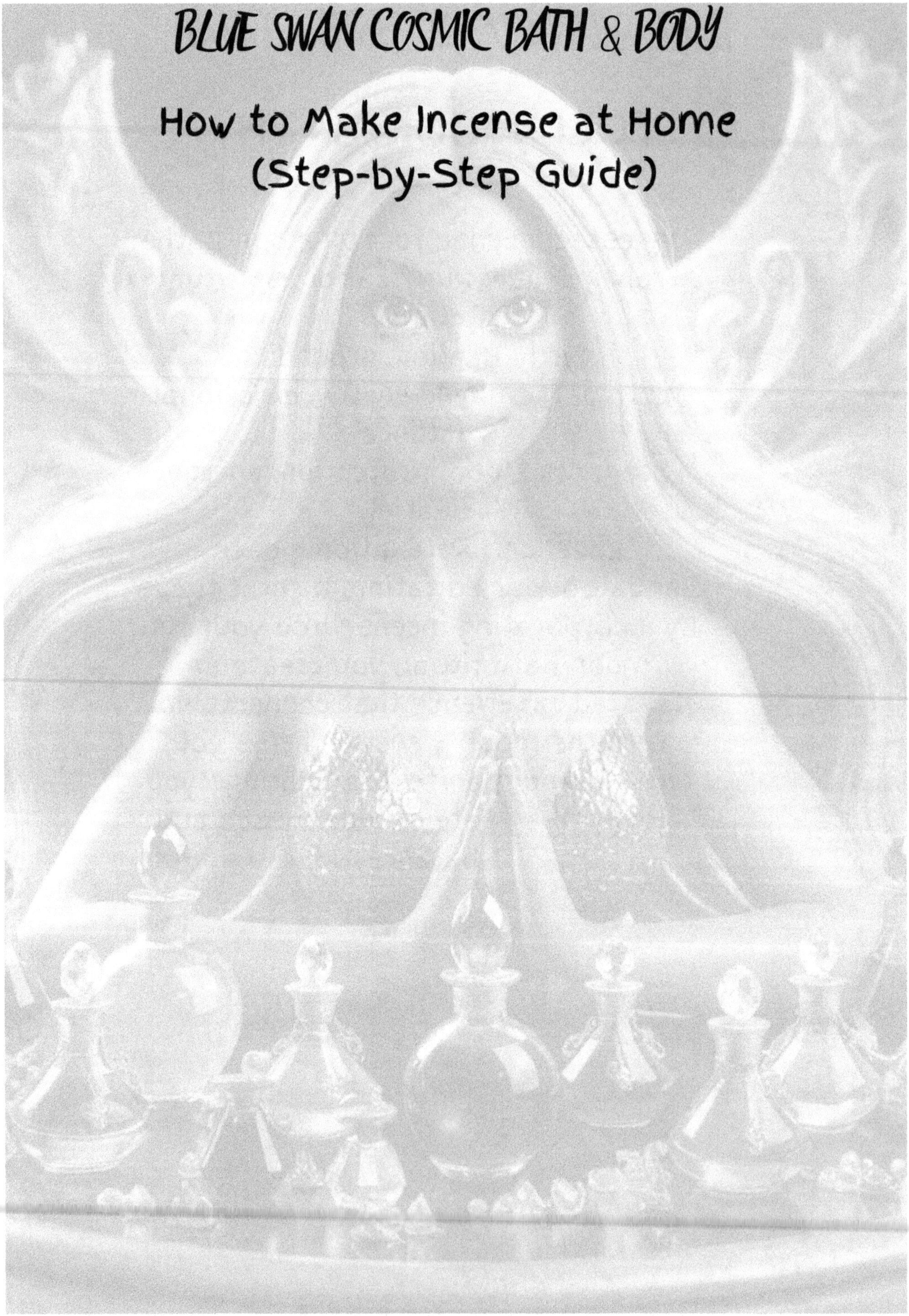

BLUE SWAN COSMIC BATH & BODY

Exotic Incense Recipes & How to Make Them
A guide to creating your own exotic incense
blends with rare, aromatic ingredients.
Incense is a great way to set the mood,
enhance meditation, or cleanse the air with
uplifting and spiritual scents.

BLUE SWAN COSMIC BATH & BODY

EXOTIC INCENSE RECIPES & HOW TO MAKE THEM

Mystic Oud & Saffron Incense

A luxurious and exotic blend with the deep, resinous notes of oud and the earthy richness of saffron.

Ingredients:

2 tablespoons Agarwood (Oud) powder (for its deep, woody, and grounding scent)

1 tablespoon Saffron threads (adds a luxurious, earthy fragrance)

1 tablespoon Frankincense resin (for its spiritual, calming aroma)

½ tablespoon Cardamom pods (for a hint of warmth and spice)

10 drops Sandalwood essential oil (for its grounding and soothing properties)

Instructions:

Grind saffron and cardamom: Use a mortar and pestle or spice grinder to finely grind the saffron threads and cardamom pods into a powder.

Combine ingredients:

Mix the ground saffron, cardamom, oud powder, and frankincense resin in a bowl.

Add essential oil:

Slowly add the sandalwood essential oil to the dry mixture, stirring continuously. It should become a slightly damp, but not too wet, paste.

Shape the incense:

If making cones, take small amounts of the mixture and shape them into cone forms with your fingers. For sticks, roll thin, even strands and gently attach them to wooden incense sticks.
Dry: Place the cones or sticks in a cool, dry place for 2-3 days to harden.

Burn and enjoy:

Once dried, burn the incense on a heat-proof dish and enjoy the exotic, luxurious aroma.

BLUE SWAN COSMIC BATH & BODY

EXOTIC INCENSE RECIPES & HOW TO MAKE THEM

Amber & Rose Exotic Incense

This blend combines the sensual and uplifting scent of roses with the deep, warming notes of amber.

Ingredients:

1 tablespoon Amber resin (for its deep, sweet, and resinous fragrance)
1 tablespoon Dried rose petals (for a sweet, floral scent)
1 tablespoon Copal resin (for its purifying and uplifting qualities)
½ tablespoon Myrrh resin (for a rich, earthy base note)
10 drops Rose essential oil (for an added boost of sweet, floral fragrance)

Instructions:

Grind the resins and petals: Use a mortar and pestle to crush the amber resin, copal, and myrrh into a fine powder. Crush the dried rose petals into smaller pieces.

Combine ingredients:

Mix all the ground ingredients in a bowl.

Add essential oil:

Slowly drizzle in the rose essential oil, stirring until the mixture forms a slightly wet, moldable consistency.

Shape the incense:

Form the mixture into cones or roll them into incense sticks as preferred.

Dry:

Allow the incense to dry in a cool place for about 2-3 days.

Use:

Once hardened, burn the incense to create an exotic, romantic ambiance.

BLUE SWAN COSMIC BATH & BODY
EXOTIC INCENSE RECIPES & HOW TO MAKE THEM

Patchouli & Vanilla Spice Incense

A warm, earthy incense blend perfect for grounding and soothing your energy.

Ingredients:

2 tablespoons Patchouli leaves (dried) (for its earthy, grounding aroma)

1 tablespoon Cinnamon powder (for a warm, spicy note)

1 tablespoon Vanilla bean powder (for a sweet, comforting aroma)

½ tablespoon Benzoin resin (for its calming, vanilla-like fragrance)

10 drops Clove essential oil (adds a layer of spice and depth)

Instructions:

Grind patchouli leaves:

Finely grind the dried patchouli leaves using a mortar and pestle or spice grinder.

Mix Ingredients:

Combine the ground patchouli, cinnamon, vanilla bean powder, and benzoin resin in a mixing bowl.

Add essential oil: Slowly incorporate the clove essential oil into the mixture, stirring continuously.

Shape into cones or sticks:

Form the paste into small cones or attach to incense sticks.

Dry for 2-3 days: Allow the incense to air dry until hardened.

Burn and enjoy:

Light and enjoy the rich, earthy scent that fills your space with warmth and comfort.

BLUE SWAN COSMIC BATH & BODY

EXOTIC INCENSE RECIPES & HOW TO MAKE THEM

Sacred Lotus & Jasmine Incense

A blend of sacred lotus and sensual jasmine, this incense is designed to uplift the spirit and promote relaxation.

Ingredients:

1 tablespoon Lotus powder (for its floral, spiritual scent)
1 tablespoon Dried jasmine flowers (for a soft, sweet floral scent)
1 tablespoon Sandalwood powder (for a grounding, earthy base)
½ tablespoon Cedarwood resin (for a slightly woody, fresh scent)
10 drops of Jasmine essential oil (for its romantic, calming properties)

Instructions:

Grind ingredients: Crush the dried jasmine flowers and cedarwood resin into a fine powder using a mortar and pestle.

Combine Ingredients:

In a bowl, mix the lotus powder, ground jasmine, sandalwood powder, and cedarwood.

Add essential oil:

Stir in the jasmine essential oil until the mixture becomes damp and moldable.

From the incense: Shape the mixture into cones or form incense sticks.

Allow to dry:

Let the incense dry for 2-3 days in a cool, dry area.

Burn:

Light your incense and enjoy the sacred, exotic scent.

BLUE SWAN COSMIC BATH & BODY
EXOTIC INCENSE RECIPES & HOW TO MAKE THEM

Cinnamon & Clove Exotic Incense

A spicy and exotic incense blend with a warming, energizing aroma.

Ingredients:

1 tablespoon Cinnamon powder (for a warm, spicy note)
1 tablespoon Clove powder (for its energizing, bold fragrance)
1 tablespoon Sandalwood powder (adds a deep, earthy base)
½ tablespoon Dried orange peel (for a bright, uplifting scent)
10 drops Orange essential oil (to enhance the citrus note)

Instructions:

Grind orange peel:

Use a mortar and pestle to grind the dried orange peel into small pieces.

Combine ingredients:

Mix the cinnamon powder, clove powder, sandalwood powder, and ground orange peel in a bowl.

Add essential oil:

Drizzle in the orange essential oil, stirring until the mixture is damp.

Shape incense:

Mold the mixture into cones or apply to sticks.

Dry the incense:

Leave the cones or sticks in a cool, dry place for 2-3 days.

Light and enjoy:

Burn the incense to fill your space with its warm, exotic spice.

BLUE SWAN COSMIC BATH & BODY

Mud and Clay Baths are a luxurious and therapeutic way to detoxify the skin, reduce inflammation, and enhance relaxation.

They have been used for centuries in beauty and wellness routines. Below are details on different types of clay, their benefits, and some bath recipes you can try.

Benefits of Mud and Clay Baths
Detoxification: Mud and clay help draw out toxins and impurities from the skin.

Skin Softening: Rich in minerals, these baths nourish and soften the skin.

Anti-inflammatory: They can soothe irritated or inflamed skin conditions like eczema, psoriasis, or acne.

Improved Circulation: Helps promote blood flow and reduce swelling.

Relaxation: The weight and texture of the mud/clay create a calming, grounding effect.

BLUE SWAN COSMIC BATH & BODY

Types of Mud and Clay

Bentonite Clay:
Rich in minerals like magnesium and calcium.
Absorbs toxins and reduces inflammation.

Rhassoul Clay:
Packed with silica, magnesium, and potassium.
Known for its moisturizing and exfoliating properties.

Dead Sea Mud:
Contains high levels of sodium, magnesium, and potassium.
Ideal for relieving skin conditions and improving elasticity.

French Green Clay:
High in iron oxide, giving it a green hue.
Best for oily or acne-prone skin, as it absorbs oils and tightens pores.

Fuller's Earth Clay:
Known for its oil-absorbing qualities.
Great for brightening the skin and clearing up blemishes.

BLUE SWAN COSMIC BATH & BODY

Mud and Clay Bath Recipes
Soothing Bentonite Clay Bath
Ingredients:
½ cup Bentonite clay
¼ cup Epsom salt
10 drops of lavender essential oil
Optional: 2 tablespoons of baking soda
Instructions:
Run a warm bath and dissolve the Epsom salts.
Mix the bentonite clay with a small amount of water to form a paste.
Add the clay paste to the bathwater and stir it around to distribute.
Add the essential oils and relax in the bath for 20-30 minutes.

BLUE SWAN COSMIC BATH & BODY

Detoxifying Dead Sea Mud Bath
Ingredients:
1 cup Dead Sea mud (you can purchase this pre-made or as a powder)
½ cup Epsom salt
5 drops eucalyptus essential oil
5 drops tea tree essential oil
Instructions:
Apply the Dead Sea mud directly onto your skin and let it sit for 10-15 minutes.
While the mud sets, run a warm bath with Epsom salts.
Once the mud is dry, rinse it off in the bath and soak for another 20 minutes, enjoying the detoxifying effects.

BLUE SWAN COSMIC BATH & BODY

French Green Clay Clarifying Bath
Ingredients:
½ cup French Green clay
¼ cup sea salt
10 drops lemongrass essential oil
5 drops peppermint essential oil
Instructions:
Run a warm bath and add the sea salt.
Mix the French Green clay with water to make a
paste and add it to the bath.
Add the essential oils and stir the water to ensure
the clay is evenly dispersed.
Relax in the bath for 20-25 minutes to allow the
clay to clarify and cleanse the skin.

BLUE SWAN COSMIC BATH & BODY

Fuller's Earth Brightening Bath
Ingredients:
½ cup Fuller's Earth clay
¼ cup Epsom salt
Juice from 1 lemon (for brightening effects)
10 drops frankincense essential oil
Instructions:
Dissolve Epsom salts in a warm bath.
Mix Fuller's Earth clay with a little water and add the lemon juice.
Add the clay mixture to the bath, along with the essential oils.
Soak for 20-30 minutes, allowing the clay to detoxify while the lemon brightens the skin.

BLUE SWAN COSMIC BATH & BODY

Enhancing the Experience
Add Flowers: Rose petals, chamomile flowers, or lavender buds can enhance the sensory experience and offer additional skin benefits.
Music: Soft, ambient music or binaural beats can help you reach deeper relaxation.
Crystals: Placing grounding crystals like black tourmaline, rose quartz, or amethyst around your bath can amplify the healing experience.
Cautions and Tips
Always do a patch test when using a new type of clay or essential oil to avoid skin irritation.
Stay hydrated by drinking water before and after your bath to support detoxification.
For a deeper detox, dry brushing before your bath helps stimulate circulation and exfoliate the skin.
Mud and clay baths offer a unique way to cleanse, restore, and rejuvenate your skin, making them perfect for luxurious self-care.

BLUE SWAN COSMIC BATH & BODY

Hydrating Rhassoul Clay and Honey Bath
Ingredients:
½ cup Rhassoul clay
2 tablespoons raw honey
10 drops rose essential oil
Optional: 1 cup full-fat milk or coconut milk
Instructions:
Mix the Rhassoul clay with honey and a bit of water to form a thick paste.
Dissolve the honey-clay mixture in a warm bath.
Add the rose oil and milk to the bathwater.
Soak for 20-30 minutes to enjoy deeply hydrated and softened skin.

BLUE SWAN COSMIC BATH & BODY

Ideal Bath Temperatures:

Warm Bath (92°F to 101°F / 33°C to 38°C):

Best for: Relaxation, soothing sore muscles, and gentle detoxification.

Benefits: This temperature helps open pores, improve circulation, and relax muscles without overstress sing the skin or cause discomfort.

Cool Bath (75°F to 90°F / 24°C to 32°C):

Best for: Reducing inflammation, boosting alertness, or recovering from physical activity.

Benefits: A cool bath can invigorate the body, reduce swelling, and is often used to soothe sunburns or relieve hot flashes.

Hot Bath (102°F to 105°F / 39°C to 40.5°C):

Best for: Deep muscle relaxation, detoxification, or cold recovery.
Caution: Prolonged hot baths can cause dehydration, dizziness, or stress on the heart. They can also dry out your skin. Limit time in a hot bath to 10-15 minutes, and avoid temperatures higher than 105°F (40.5°C).

Factors to Consider:

Personal Comfort: Always prioritize your comfort. If the water feels too hot or too cold, adjust it to what feels best for your body.

Skin Sensitivity:

If you have sensitive or dry skin, it's best to stick to warm baths (around 95°F to 98°F) to avoid irritation or dehydration.

Health Conditions:

If you have certain health conditions, such as cardiovascular issues, it's important to consult with a healthcare professional about the appropriate bath temperature for you.
For most people, a warm bath around 98°F (37°C), which is close to body temperature, offers the most benefits without any discomfort, making it the perfect balance for relaxation and skin health.

BLUE SWAN COSMIC BATH & BODY

The *ideal bath temperature for relaxation, skin health, and overall well-being* typically falls between 92°F to 101°F (33°C to 38°C). This temperature range is considered "warm" and offers a soothing, relaxing experience without being too hot, which can cause dehydration or stress to the skin.

Here's how different bath temperatures can impact your experience:

Making bath bombs at home is a fun and easy DIY project. Bath bombs are a delightful addition to your bathing routine, providing fizz, color, and fragrance.

Here's a simple recipe along with variations and tips for creating your own bath bombs.

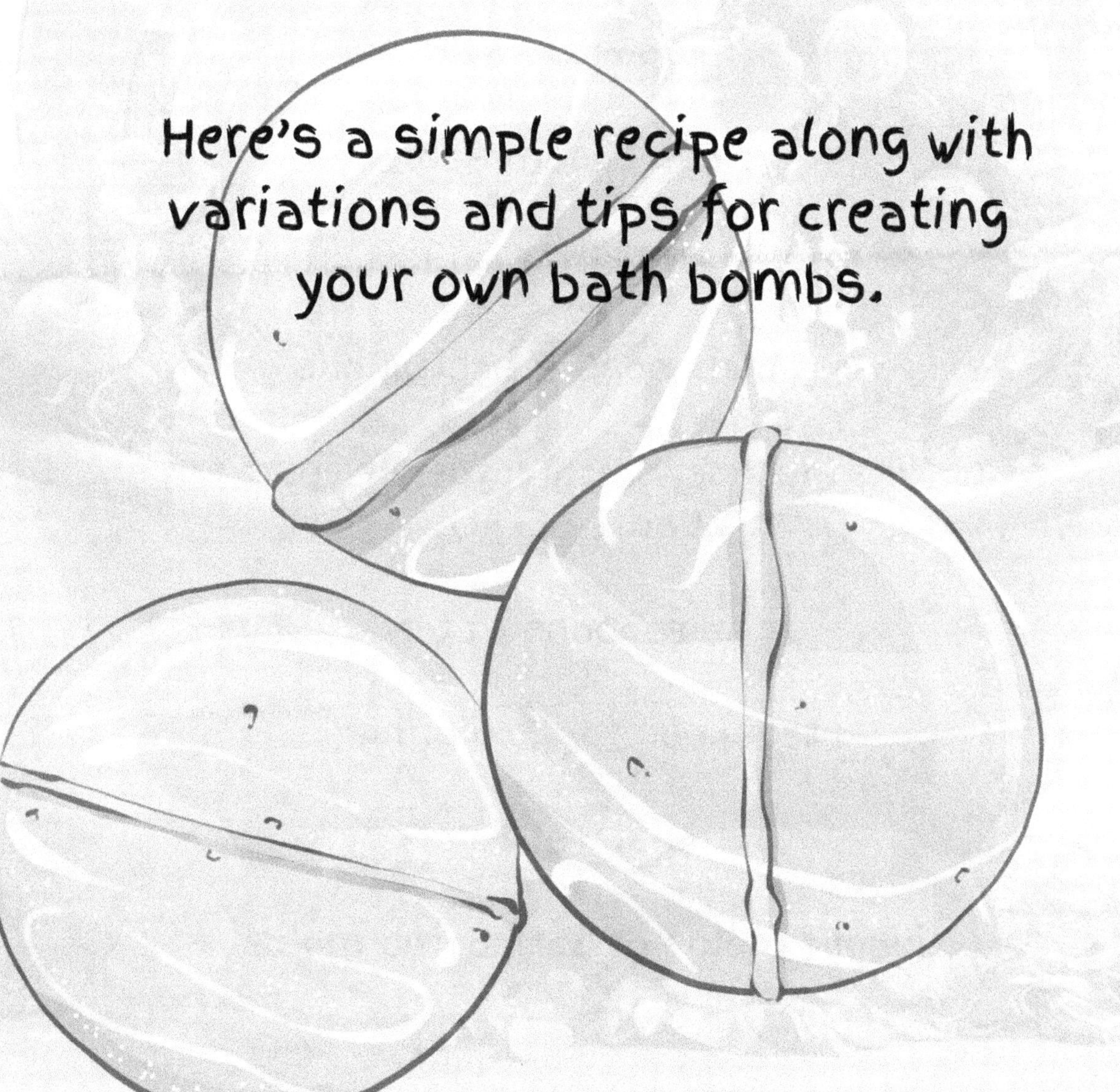

BLUE SWAN COSMIC BATH & BODY

HOW TO MAKE BATH BOMBS

Basic Bath Bomb Recipe

Ingredients:

1 cup baking soda

1/2 cup citric acid

1/2 cup Epsom salt

1/2 cup citric acid

2 1/2 tablespoons essential oils

(like lavender, eucalyptus, or your favorite scent)

2 tablespoons water

1 teaspoon food coloring

(optional, for color)

Silicone molds or bath bomb molds

BLUE SWAN COSMIC BATH & BODY
HOW TO MAKE BATH BOMBS
Variations

Colorful Bath Bombs:

Use different food colorings for vibrant bath bombs. You can divide the mixture into multiple bowls and color each part differently.

Herbal Infusions:
Add dried herbs (like lavender, chamomile, or rose petals) to your mixture for added benefits and a lovely aesthetic.

Milk Powder Bath Bombs:
Incorporate powdered milk (like goat milk or coconut milk) for extra moisture in the bath.

Scented Bath Bombs:
Experiment with various essential oils such as peppermint, jasmine, or eucalyptus to create unique scents.

Coconut Oil Bath Bombs:
Substitute the water with melted coconut oil for added hydration.

BLUE SWAN COSMIC BATH & BODY

HOW TO MAKE BATH BOMBS

Tips for Success
Don't Overmix: Be careful not to overmix your ingredients, as this can cause them to fizz prematurely.

Storage:
Store your bath bombs in a cool, dry place away from moisture to prevent them from activating before use.

Testing:
Test a small batch first to refine your method and ratios before making larger quantities.

Cleaning Up:
If you're using food coloring, be cautious as it can stain surfaces. Consider using a bowl that you don't mind staining, or wear gloves.

BLUE SWAN COSMIC BATH & BODY

HOW TO MAKE BATH BOMBS

How to Use Bath Bombs

Fill the Tub:
Start filling your bathtub with warm water.

Drop in the Bath Bomb:
Once the tub is filled, drop the bath bomb
in and watch it fizz and dissolve.

Enjoy:
Soak in the aromatic, colorful water for a
relaxing experience.

Troubleshooting Common Issues

Bath Bombs Crumble:
If your bath bombs are crumbling, they may
have been too dry. Try adding a tiny bit more
liquid next time.

Bath Bombs Don't Fizz:
If your bath bombs don't fizz, it could be due
to moisture exposure during storage.

Keep them in a dry place until use.

Now you're all set to create your own beautiful
and fragrant bath bombs at home! Enjoy your
relaxing bath experience!

BLUE SWAN COSMIC BATH & BODY
FRUITS TO ADD TO YOUR BATH

Bathing in fruit juice is a practice that has been used for centuries by various cultures, often associated with beauty rituals, health benefits, and spiritual significance. Here's a closer look at this intriguing practice and its cultural context:

BLUE SWAN COSMIC BATH & BODY
FRUITS TO ADD TO YOUR BATH

Ancient Civilizations:

Many ancient civilizations, such as the Egyptians, Greeks, and Romans, recognized the benefits of fruit and their juices for skin health. They would often use natural ingredients in their bathing practices, incorporating fruits known for their beneficial properties.

Beauty Rituals:

In some cultures, fruit juices were believed to enhance beauty. For example, Cleopatra was famously known to bathe in milk and honey, but other fruits like pomegranates, figs, and grapes were also used for their rich vitamins and antioxidants, which were thought to promote radiant skin.

Cultural Practices:

In many indigenous cultures, fruit juices and pulps were used in ceremonial baths to purify the body and spirit. These rituals often included prayers or intentions for healing, beauty, and connection to nature.

BLUE SWAN COSMIC BATH & BODY

BENEFITS OF BATHING IN FRUIT JUICE

Nourishment for Skin:

Many fruits are rich in vitamins (like C and E), antioxidants, and natural acids that can help exfoliate, hydrate, and brighten the skin. For example, citrus juices (like lemon and orange) can help in natural exfoliation, while others like avocado and banana can provide deep hydration.

Aromatherapy:

The natural fragrances of fruits can enhance relaxation and create a calming atmosphere. The scents from fruit juices can uplift mood and relieve stress during bathing.

Cultural Significance:

For some women, bathing in fruit juice is more than just a beauty ritual; it can be a form of self-care, a way to connect with their heritage, or a spiritual practice.

BLUE SWAN COSMIC BATH & BODY

FRUITS TO ADD TO YOUR BATH

Modern Interpretations

In contemporary wellness and spa practices, bathing in fruit juice has seen a resurgence, often as part of luxurious spa treatments or at-home self-care rituals. Here are some examples:

Spa Treatments:

Many high-end spas offer fruit-infused baths as part of their treatment menu. These baths often include a combination of fruit juices, essential oils, and therapeutic salts to enhance skin benefits and relaxation.

DIY Rituals:

Women may create their own fruit juice baths at home using fresh, organic juices or pulps. Ingredients like coconut milk, aloe vera, and various fruit juices can be blended into bathwater for a nourishing soak.

Social Media Trends:

Platforms like Instagram and TikTok have popularized unique bath experiences, including fruit juice baths. Many women share their rituals, showcasing the vibrant colors and textures of fruit juices in their baths, inspiring others to explore self-care through nature.

BLUE SWAN COSMIC BATH & BODY
FRUITS TO ADD TO YOUR BATH

The practice of bathing in fruit juice embodies a blend of historical significance, beauty rituals, and modern wellness trends.

Whether as a luxurious treat at a spa or a personal self-care ritual at home, it connects women with nature and offers nourishment for both the body and spirit.

Embracing such practices can enhance the overall bathing experience, making it not just a routine but a sacred time for reflection and rejuvenation.

BLUE SWAN COSMIC BATH & BODY
FRUITY BATH RECIPE

Ingredients:
1 cup Epsom salt
1 cup sea salt or Himalayan salt
1 cup baking soda
1 cup citric acid
1 cup dried flowers or herbs (such as lavender, chamomile, or rose petals)
1-2 cups of fresh fruit (sliced; options include strawberries, oranges, lemons, or cucumbers)
2-3 tablespoons essential oils (such as lemon, orange, or lavender)
Optional: A few drops of food coloring (natural colors work best)
Optional: A few drops of natural oils (like coconut or olive oil) for added moisture

Instructions:

Prepare the Fruit:
Slice your chosen fresh fruit into thin rounds or quarters. You can use a mix of fruits for variety and color.

Mix the Dry Ingredients:
In a large mixing bowl, combine the Epsom salt, sea salt, baking soda, citric acid, and dried flowers or herbs. Mix well to ensure everything is evenly distributed.

Add Essential Oils:
Add the essential oils to the dry mixture, stirring well to combine. If you're using food coloring, add it here and mix until the color is evenly distributed.

Add the Fresh Fruit:
Gently fold the sliced fruit into the mixture. The fruit can also be added directly to the bath for extra visual appeal.

Package the Bath Mix:
Transfer the fruit bath mixture into an airtight container or a glass jar. It can be used immediately or stored for future use.

BLUE SWAN COSMIC BATH & BODY
FRUITS TO ADD TO YOUR BATH

How to Use the Fruit Bath Mixture:
Fill Your Tub:
Fill your bathtub with warm water.
Add the Bath Mix:
Pour in your fruit bath mixture. You can also toss the sliced fruit into the tub for a beautiful presentation.
Soak and Enjoy:
Relax in the fruity bath for at least 20-30 minutes, allowing the Epsom salt and essential oils to work their magic on your skin.
Clean Up:
After your bath, rinse off to remove any remaining salt or fruit residue. Consider using a strainer to catch any bits of fruit before draining the tub.
Benefits of a Fruit Bath:
Exfoliation: The natural acids in fruits like lemons and oranges can help exfoliate the skin, leaving it smooth and radiant.
Hydration:
Ingredients like coconut oil can help hydrate and nourish the skin.
Aromatherapy:
The essential oils from the fruits and additional oils promote relaxation and enhance your mood.

Visual Appeal:
The colors and shapes of the fruit create a beautiful, inviting bath experience.
Feel free to experiment with different fruit combinations and essential oils to create your perfect fruity bath recipe! Enjoy your luxurious soak!

BLUE SWAN COSMIC BATH & BODY
FRUITS TO ADD TO YOUR BATH

Lemon:
Benefits: Brightening and refreshing, lemon can help invigorate your senses. Its natural acidity may help exfoliate and brighten the skin.

Orange:
Benefits: Similar to lemon, orange provides a zesty aroma and uplifting scent. The vitamin C in oranges can help nourish the skin.

Strawberries:
Benefits: Rich in antioxidants, strawberries can help brighten the skin and provide hydration. They also add a lovely color and fragrance.

Cucumber:
Benefits: Known for its soothing and hydrating properties, cucumber can help cool the skin and reduce puffiness.

Avocado:
Benefits: Packed with healthy fats, avocado can moisturize and nourish the skin. Its creamy texture can enhance the luxurious feel of your bath.

Raspberries:
Benefits: High in antioxidants and vitamins, raspberries can help rejuvenate the skin and provide a natural glow.

Peaches:
Benefits: The natural sugars in peaches can help moisturize and soften the skin, while their fragrance is sweet and inviting.

BLUE SWAN COSMIC BATH & BODY
FRUITS TO ADD TO YOUR BATH

Pineapple:
Benefits: Rich in bromelain, pineapple can help exfoliate dead skin cells and promote a healthy complexion.

Watermelon:
Benefits: Hydrating and refreshing, watermelon is great for soothing the skin and keeping it cool during warm baths.

Blueberries:
Benefits: These tiny fruits are packed with antioxidants and can help protect the skin from free radical damage.

Banana:
Benefits: The natural oils in bananas can help moisturize the skin, making it soft and smooth.

Grapefruit:
Benefits: Its refreshing scent and natural astringent properties can help tone the skin and invigorate your senses.

Mango:
Benefits: Rich in vitamins A and C, mango can nourish and brighten the skin while adding a tropical fragrance to your bath.

Pomegranate:
Benefits: Known for its high antioxidant content, pomegranate can help rejuvenate the skin and promote a youthful appearance.

BLUE SWAN COSMIC BATH & BODY
FRUITS TO ADD TO YOUR BATH

Tips for Using Fruits in Your Bath

Preparation:
Wash and slice the fruits into thin pieces or wedges for better infusion in the bathwater.

Direct Use:
You can toss whole fruits or slices directly into the tub for a colorful display.

Infusion Bags:
Consider placing sliced fruits in a muslin bag or cheesecloth to prevent pieces from floating around, making cleanup easier.

Combine with Other Ingredients:
Mix fruits with bath salts, essential oils, or herbs for a more aromatic and beneficial experience.

Adding these fruits to your bath can create a rejuvenating and sensory-rich experience, enhancing your relaxation while providing skin benefits! Enjoy your fruity bath!

BLUE SWAN COSMIC BATH & BODY

BENEFITS OF MILK BATHS

Milk baths have been celebrated for their skin-soothing and beautifying properties for centuries.

This ancient practice is still cherished today for its numerous benefits. Here's an overview of milk baths, their historical significance, benefits, how to create one, and tips for enhancing the experience:

Historical Significance

Ancient Beauty Rituals:

Cleopatra, the famed queen of Egypt, is famously known for her milk baths, believing they contributed to her legendary beauty. The practice dates back to ancient civilizations, where milk was used not only for nourishment but also as a luxurious skin treatment.

Cultural Practices:

Various cultures around the world have incorporated milk into their bathing rituals. For instance, in India, milk is often used in traditional Ayurvedic practices for its healing properties.

BLUE SWAN COSMIC BATH & BODY

BENEFITS OF MILK BATHS

Moisturization:

Milk contains fats and proteins that help to hydrate and nourish the skin. It can leave the skin feeling soft and supple.

Exfoliation:

Lactic acid, found in milk, is a natural alpha-hydroxy acid (AHA) that helps exfoliate dead skin cells, promoting a smoother and brighter complexion.

Soothing Properties:

Milk baths can be especially beneficial for sensitive or irritated skin. The proteins in milk can help soothe inflammation and redness.

Anti-Aging:

The antioxidants in milk can help combat signs of aging, such as dryness and fine lines, giving the skin a youthful glow.

Relaxation:

The warm milk combined with soothing scents can create a calming atmosphere, making milk baths an excellent way to unwind and de-stress.

BLUE SWAN COSMIC BATH & BODY

HOW TO CREATE A MILK BATH

How to Create a Milk Bath

Ingredients:
Milk:
You can use whole milk, powdered milk, or even coconut milk for a dairy-free option.

Optional Additives:
Essential oils (like lavender or chamomile for relaxation)
Honey (for extra hydration)
Oats (for additional soothing properties)
Epsom salt (for muscle relaxation)

Instructions:
Prepare the Bath:
Fill your tub with warm water (not too hot, as this can be drying to the skin).

Add Milk:
Pour in about 2 cups of whole milk or powdered milk (mixed with warm water) into the tub.

Incorporate Additives:
If using, add a few drops of essential oils, honey, or oats to enhance the bath experience.

Soak:
Relax in the milk bath for about 15-20 minutes to allow your skin to absorb the nourishing properties.

Rinse Off:
After soaking, rinse your body with warm water to remove any residue.

BLUE SWAN COSMIC BATH & BODY
BEST HERBS FOR MILK BATHS

Lavender:
Benefits: Known for its calming properties, lavender can help reduce stress and anxiety while promoting relaxation. It has antiseptic qualities that can benefit the skin.
How to Use: Use dried lavender buds or lavender essential oil.

Chamomile:
Benefits: Chamomile is soothing and can help calm irritated skin. It also has anti-inflammatory properties, making it great for sensitive skin.
How to Use: Add dried chamomile flowers or chamomile essential oil.

Rose Petals:
Benefits: Rose petals are not only beautiful but also help hydrate and rejuvenate the skin. Their scent is uplifting and promotes a feeling of romance and relaxation.
How to Use: Use fresh or dried rose petals in the bath.

Oat Straw:
Benefits: Oat straw is known for its skin-soothing properties and can help alleviate dryness and irritation. It's especially beneficial for sensitive skin.
How to Use: Use dried oat straw or oat extract.

Calendula:
Benefits: Calendula has healing properties and can help soothe inflamed or irritated skin. It's great for conditions like eczema and dermatitis.
How to Use: Add dried calendula flowers to the milk bath.

BLUE SWAN COSMIC BATH & BODY

BEST HERBS FOR MILK BATHS

Peppermint:
Benefits: The cooling effect of peppermint can be invigorating and refreshing. It can also help relieve muscle tension and headaches.
How to Use: Use dried peppermint leaves or peppermint essential oil.

Hibiscus:
Benefits: Hibiscus is rich in antioxidants and vitamins, which can help brighten and nourish the skin. It also has natural exfoliating properties.
How to Use: Add dried hibiscus petals or hibiscus tea to the bath.

Sage:
Benefits: Sage has antibacterial properties and can help cleanse the skin. Its earthy scent can also promote relaxation and clarity of mind.
How to Use: Use dried sage leaves or sage essential oil.

Thyme:
Benefits: Thyme is rich in antioxidants and has antimicrobial properties, which can help keep the skin healthy. Its aroma can also promote relaxation.
How to Use: Use dried thyme leaves or thyme essential oil.

Lemon Balm:
Benefits: Lemon balm is soothing and can help calm the mind. Its citrusy scent is refreshing and uplifting.
How to Use: Use dried lemon balm leaves or lemon balm essential oil.

BLUE SWAN COSMIC BATH & BODY

TIPS

FOR ENHANCING YOUR MILK BATH EXPERIENCE

Set the Ambiance:

Dim the lights or use candles for a calming atmosphere. Soft music or nature sounds can enhance relaxation.

Add Fruits:

For added luxury, consider floating slices of fruits like lemons, oranges, or strawberries in the bath.

Use a Bath Tray:

Place a tray over the tub to hold a book, a glass of herbal tea, or your favorite snacks to enjoy while you soak.

Incorporate Aromatherapy:

Use essential oils in a diffuser nearby to create a soothing scent in the air.

Follow Up with Moisturizer:

After your milk bath, apply a good moisturizer to lock in hydration.

BLUE SWAN COSMIC BATH & BODY

MILK BATHS

Milk baths offer a timeless and luxurious way to pamper yourself while providing numerous skin benefits.

Whether you're seeking relaxation, hydration, or a touch of historical beauty ritual, a milk bath can be a delightful addition to your self-care routine.

Embrace the soothing qualities of milk and enjoy a rejuvenating bathing experience!
40 mini

BLUE SWAN COSMIC BATH & BODY
BATH RITUALS

Full Moon Ritual Bath

Ingredients:

Epsom salts
Lavender essential oil
Fresh or dried chamomile
Rose petals
A white candle for purification
A crystal (like clear quartz or moonstone) to amplify
energy

Instructions:
Prepare Your Space: Light the candle and arrange the
crystal nearby. Fill the tub with warm water.

Add Ingredients:
Sprinkle in Epsom salts, a few drops of lavender oil,
chamomile, and rose petals while focusing on your
intention for the bath.

Meditation:
As you soak, meditate on your intentions for the full
moon, visualizing release and renewal.
Gratitude: Conclude your ritual by expressing gratitude for
the lessons learned during the moon cycle.

BLUE SWAN COSMIC BATH & BODY

BATH RITUALS

Detox Bath Ritual

Ingredients:

Baking soda
Apple cider vinegar
Sea salt or Himalayan pink salt
Fresh ginger or ginger essential oil
A soothing tea (like peppermint or green tea)

Instructions:

Prepare the Bath:
Fill the tub with warm water and add baking soda, sea salt, and apple cider vinegar.

Add Ginger:
Grate fresh ginger into the bath or add a few drops of ginger oil for a warming effect.

Relax and Detox:
Soak for 20-30 minutes, sipping on your herbal tea to stay hydrated.

Post-Bath Routine:
Rinse off with cool water to close the pores and help flush out toxins.

BLUE SWAN COSMIC BATH & BODY

BATH RITUALS

Luxury Spa Bath Ritual

Ingredients:

Organic coconut milk
Honey
Essential oils (like vanilla or sandalwood)
Fresh fruit slices (like oranges or strawberries)
Soft music or nature sounds

Instructions:

Create a Spa Atmosphere:
Dim the lights and play calming music. Fill the tub with warm water.

Mix Your Ingredients:
Blend coconut milk and honey, then pour into t

Add Fruit:
Float fresh fruit slices on the water's surface for a refreshing touch.

Indulge:
Soak for 30-45 minutes, focusing on relaxation and self-love.

BLUE SWAN COSMIC BATH & BODY

BATH RITUALS

Healing Crystal Bath Ritual

Ingredients:

Epsom salts

Your favorite essential oils (like frankincense or rose)
Healing crystals (like amethyst, rose quartz, or citrine)

Instructions:

Set Your Intention: Before starting the bath, meditate on what healing you seek (physical, emotional, or spiritual).

Prepare the Bath:

Fill the tub with warm water and add Epsom salts and a few drops of your chosen essential oils.

Place Crystals:

Set your chosen healing crystals around the tub or in the water (if safe) to enhance the energy.

Relax and Visualize:

As you soak, visualize healing energy flowing through your body and releasing any negativity.

BLUE SWAN COSMIC BATH & BODY
BATH RITUALS

Fruit & Milk Bath Ritual

Ingredients:

Whole milk or coconut milk
Fresh fruits (like strawberries, oranges, or kiwi)
Honey

Instructions:

Prepare the Milk Bath:

Fill the tub with warm water and add whole milk or
coconut milk for a creamy texture.

Add Fruits:
Slice fresh fruits and add them to the bath for a
fragrant and luxurious touch.

Sweeten the Deal:
Drizzle honey into the bath for added moisture
and nourishment for the skin.

Enjoy the Experience:
Relax for 30 minutes, allowing the milk and fruits
to hydrate and soothe your skin.

BLUE SWAN COSMIC BATH & BODY

BATH RITUALS

Candle and Incense Bath Ritual

Ingredients:

Scented candles
(lavender, sandalwood)
Incense sticks
(frankincense, myrrh, or any preferred scent)

Bath salts or oils

Instructions:

Create Ambiance:

Light candles and incense before running the bath to
set the mood.

Fill the Tub:

Add bath salts or oils while the water is running.
Soak and Breathe: As you relax in the bath, focus on
the soothing scents and calming atmosphere. Take
deep breaths to enhance relaxation.

Mindfulness:

Spend this time in mindfulness or prayer, allowing the
scents to transport you to a peaceful state.

BLUE SWAN COSMIC BATH & BODY

BATH RITUALS

Incorporating these bath rituals into your routine can provide a multi-sensory experience that promotes relaxation, healing, and rejuvenation.

Feel free to mix and match elements from different rituals to create a personalized experience that resonates with your needs and desires.

Enjoy your luxurious bathing journey!

BLUE SWAN COSMIC BATH & BODY

Praying in the bath can be a beautiful way to combine self-care with spiritual practice, creating a serene environment to connect with your inner self or a higher power.

Here's how to pray in the bath and some recommendations for candles to enhance your experience.

BLUE SWAN COSMIC BATH & BODY

BATH PRAYERS

Prayer for Peace "As I soak in this warm bath, I invite peace to flow through me. May the worries of the day dissolve like the salts in this water. I release all negativity and embrace tranquility. Thank you, Divine Mother, for this moment of serenity."

Prayer for Healing "With each drop of water that touches my skin, I call upon healing energy to fill my body. I release any pain, stress, or burden, and I welcome health and vitality. May this bath restore my spirit and renew my strength."

Prayer of Gratitude "I am grateful for this time to nurture myself. Thank you for the warmth of this water, the scents that surround me, and the opportunity to relax. I acknowledge my worthiness and honor my journey with love and gratitude."

Prayer for Self-Love "In this sacred space, I embrace my true self. I let go of self-doubt and open my heart to love and acceptance. I am worthy of joy, peace, and happiness. May this bath remind me of my beauty and strength."

Prayer for Clarity "As I immerse myself in this water, I seek clarity and insight. May this time of reflection bring me wisdom and guidance. I trust in the process and know that I am on the right path. Thank you for the light that guides me."

BLUE SWAN COSMIC BATH & BODY
POSITIVE AFFIRMATIONS

"I am deserving of love and peace."

"Every drop of water nourishes my mind, body, and spirit."

"I release all negativity and embrace positivity."

"I am in tune with my inner self and trust my intuition."

"I honor my body and treat it with kindness and respect."

"I am capable of overcoming any challenges that come my way."

"I radiate confidence and grace."

"I am surrounded by love and support."

"My mind is clear, and my heart is open."

"I attract abundance and joy into my life."

Feel free to recite these prayers and affirmations before or during your bath to enhance your experience and cultivate a sense of peace and self-empowerment.

Enjoy your time of relaxation and self-care!

BLUE SWAN COSMIC BATH & BODY

BATH RITUALS

Herbal Tea Bath Ritual

Ingredients:

Herbal tea bags (like chamomile, lavender, or green tea)
A muslin bag or tea infuser
Honey or sugar (for exfoliation)

Instructions:

Brew Herbal Tea: Steep several tea bags in hot water to create a strong herbal infusion.

Prepare the Bath:

Add the herbal infusion to the bathwater along with any additional ingredients like honey for skin benefits.

Soak and Exfoliate:

While soaking, gently scrub your skin with sugar or honey to exfoliate.

Reflect:

Use this time for reflection or journaling about your feelings and thoughts.

BLUE SWAN COSMIC BATH & BODY

CRYSTALS

Tips for Using Crystals in the Bath:

Cleanse the Crystals:
Before using them, cleanse your crystals to remove any negative energy. You can do this by rinsing them under running water, placing them in sunlight, or using sage smoke.

Use a Pouch:
If you're concerned about debris or dirt from the crystals, consider placing them in a muslin bag or cheesecloth before adding them to your bath.

Infuse Crystal Water:
You can also make crystal-infused water by placing the stones in a jar of water and letting it sit for several hours. Add this infused water to your bath.

Always ensure that the crystals you use are safe for water exposure, as some can be damaged by water or may leach harmful substances. Enjoy your soothing and energetically charged bath!

BLUE SWAN COSMIC BATH & BODY

CRYSTALS

Using crystals in your bath can enhance the experience, bringing various benefits depending on the type of crystal you choose.

Here are some popular crystals to consider for your bath:

BLUE SWAN COSMIC BATH & BODY

CRYSTALS

Amethyst
Benefits: Promotes calmness and balance, enhances intuition, and encourages restful sleep.
How to Use: Place a few polished amethyst stones in your bath or a sachet filled with amethyst chips.

Rose Quartz
Benefits: Known as the stone of love, it promotes self-love, compassion, and emotional healing.
How to Use: Add rose quartz to your bath or use rose quartz oil infused with its energy.

Clear Quartz
Benefits: Known for its amplifying properties, it can enhance energy and intentions, promoting clarity and healing.
How to Use: Place clear quartz crystals around the bath or in a pouch in the water.

Citrine
Benefits: Known for attracting abundance and joy, it can uplift your mood and stimulate creativity.
How to Use: Use citrine crystals in the bath to soak up positive energy and joy.

Selenite
Benefits: Provides a calming effect and can help with mental clarity, purification, and spiritual connection.
How to Use: Place selenite sticks on the edge of the tub or use selenite-infused water.

BLUE SWAN COSMIC BATH & BODY

CRYSTALS

Selenite

Benefits: Provides a calming effect and can help with mental clarity, purification, and spiritual connection.
How to Use: Place selenite sticks on the edge of the tub or use selenite-infused water.

Black Tourmaline

Benefits: Offers protection from negative energy, grounding, and emotional stability.
How to Use: Place black tourmaline in your bath to help dispel negativity.

Lapis Lazuli

Benefits: Encourages self-awareness and self-expression, promoting inner truth and wisdom.
How to Use: Use lapis lazuli stones in your bath for enhanced communication and clarity.

Jade

Benefits: Known for its soothing and healing properties, it promotes balance and harmony.
How to Use: Add jade stones or a jade roller to your bath for a refreshing experience.

Carnelian

Benefits: Boosts motivation, creativity, and confidence, and helps with emotional balance.
How to Use: Place carnelian stones in the bath to ignite your passion and creativity.

Moonstone

Benefits: Enhances intuition and emotional balance, often associated with feminine energy and new beginnings.
How to Use: Use moonstone in your bath to connect with your inner self and the moon's energy.

BLUE SWAN COSMIC BATH & BODY

BATH SNACKS
IDEAS AND RECIPES

Tips for Enjoying Snacks in the Bath:

Use a Tray:
Consider using a bath tray to hold your snacks and drinks, keeping everything within reach and safe from splashes.

Keep It Simple:
Choose snacks that are easy to eat and won't make a mess. Avoid anything too sticky or crumbly.

Hydration:
Don't forget to hydrate! Keep a glass of water, herbal tea, or infused water nearby to sip on while you relax.

Indulging in these snacks while enjoying a luxurious bath can elevate your self-care routine and make it even more delightful!

BLUE SWAN COSMIC BATH & BODY
Bath SNACKS
IDEAS AND RECIPES

Fruit Skewers
Ingredients: Fresh fruits like strawberries, pineapple, grapes, and melon.
Preparation:
Cut the fruits into bite-sized pieces and thread them onto skewers for easy eating. The sweetness of the fruits will complement your bath experience.

Chocolate-Covered Strawberries
Ingredients: Fresh strawberries and dark or milk chocolate.
Preparation: Melt chocolate, dip strawberries, and let them cool on parchment paper. These are a luxurious treat that feels special.

Cheese and Crackers
Ingredients: A selection of your favorite cheeses and crackers.
Preparation: Arrange cheese slices or cubes with assorted crackers on a plate. Pair with some grapes or nuts for added flavor.

Veggies and Hummus
Ingredients: Fresh vegetables like carrots, celery, cucumber, and bell peppers with hummus.

Preparation:
Slice the veggies and serve with a small bowl of hummus for dipping. This snack is healthy and refreshing.

Nuts and Dried Fruits
Ingredients: A mix of your favorite nuts (almonds, cashews, walnuts) and dried fruits (raisins, cranberries, apricots).
Preparation: Combine nuts and dried fruits in a small bowl for a nutritious and satisfying snack.

Dark Chocolate Squares
Ingredients: High-quality dark chocolate.
Preparation: Keep some dark chocolate squares nearby for a decadent treat that pairs well with relaxation.

Granola Bars
Ingredients: Homemade or store-bought granola bars.
Preparation: Pack a few granola bars to munch on while you soak. They provide energy and taste great.

Coconut Chips
Ingredients: Unsweetened coconut chips.
Preparation: Enjoy the crunchy texture of coconut chips. They offer a tropical twist and are perfect for snacking.

Smoothie Bowl
Ingredients: Blend your favorite fruits with yogurt or milk, and top with granola, nuts, and seeds.

Preparation:
Make a smoothie bowl to enjoy before or after your bath. Use a wide bowl for easy access while lounging.

BLUE SWAN COSMIC BATH & BODY
Bath SNACKS
IDEAS AND RECIPES

Chocolate-Covered Bananas
Ingredients:
1 ripe banana
1 cup dark chocolate chips
Sea salt (optional)
Instructions:
Slice the banana into bite-sized pieces.
Melt the chocolate chips in the microwave in 30-second
intervals, stirring until smooth.
Dip each banana piece in the melted chocolate and place
them on parchment paper.
Sprinkle with a pinch of sea salt if desired.
Freeze for about 15-20 minutes until the chocolate hardens.

Fruit & Yogurt Parfait
Ingredients:
1 cup Greek yogurt (plain or flavored)
1 cup mixed fresh berries (strawberries, blueberries,
raspberries)
2 tablespoons granola or nuts
Instructions:
In a glass or bowl, layer half of the yogurt at the bottom.
Add a layer of fresh berries and sprinkle with granola or
nuts.
Repeat the layers until all ingredients are used.
Enjoy right away!

Cinnamon Apple Chips
Ingredients:
1 apple (any variety)
1 teaspoon cinnamon
1 tablespoon sugar (optional)
Instructions:
Preheat your oven to 200°F (95°C).
Core and thinly slice the apple.
Arrange the apple slices on a baking sheet lined with
parchment paper.
Sprinkle cinnamon (and sugar, if using) evenly over the apple
slices.
Bake for 1-2 hours until crispy, flipping halfway through.
Let cool and enjoy!

BLUE SWAN COSMIC BATH & BODY
Bath SNACKS
IDEAS AND RECIPES

Peanut Butter & Celery Sticks
Ingredients:
2 celery stalks
2 tablespoons peanut butter
Raisins or chocolate chips (optional)
Instructions:
Wash and cut the celery stalks into 3-4 inch pieces.
Spread peanut butter into the groove of each celery stick.
Top with raisins or chocolate chips for added sweetness.
Enjoy as a crunchy, satisfying snack!

Mini Caprese Skewers
Ingredients:
Cherry tomatoes
Fresh mozzarella balls (bocconcini)
Fresh basil leaves
Balsamic glaze (optional)
Salt and pepper (to taste)
Instructions:
On toothpicks or small skewers, thread a cherry tomato, a basil leaf, and a mozzarella ball.
Repeat until all ingredients are used.
Drizzle with balsamic glaze and sprinkle with salt and pepper before serving.
These quick recipes are perfect for snacking while you unwind in the bath. Enjoy your relaxation time!
40 mini

BLUE SWAN COSMIC BATH & BODY
USE FREQUENCIES DURING BATHING

How to Use Frequencies During Bathing:

Speakers or Waterproof Devices:
Play these frequencies through speakers or a waterproof device while you soak.

Meditation Apps:
Use binaural beats apps that allow you to choose specific frequencies and create customized soundscapes for your bath.

Combine with Aromatherapy:
Enhance the experience by lighting candles, using essential oils, or adding bath salts that complement the emotional or physical benefits of the chosen frequency.

Incorporating these sounds into your water bathing routine can elevate the sensory experience, offering deep relaxation, healing, and emotional cleansing.

BLUE SWAN COSMIC BATH & BODY
USE FREQUENCIES DURING BATHING

Binaural beats and specific sound frequencies can enhance your bathing experience by promoting relaxation, healing, and mental clarity.

Here are some of the best frequencies and binaural sounds to incorporate during water bathing:

BLUE SWAN COSMIC BATH & BODY
USE FREQUENCIES DURING BATHING

432 Hz – The Frequency of Nature

Benefits: Known as the "natural tuning" frequency, 432 Hz is said to resonate with the universe's vibrations, bringing a sense of harmony, relaxation, and inner peace.

Use in Bathing:

This frequency can help align your body's energy with nature and create a calming atmosphere, making it perfect for a deeply soothing bath.

528 Hz – The Love Frequency

Benefits: Often called the "miracle tone" or "DNA repair frequency," 528 Hz is believed to heal and promote love, harmony, and balance. Use in Bathing: This is ideal for emotional healing and self-love rituals in the bath, helping you release negative emotions and focus on self-care.

396 Hz – Liberation from Fear

Benefits: This frequency helps release feelings of fear, guilt, and anxiety, promoting emotional liberation.

Use in Bathing:

Perfect for a detox bath, helping you let go of emotional blocks while cleansing your body and mind.

639 Hz – Harmonizing Relationships

Benefits: Known to balance and harmonize relationships, this frequency fosters connection, love, and compassion.

Use in Bathing:

Great for meditative baths focused on improving your relationship with yourself or others, enhancing feelings of connectedness.

BLUE SWAN COSMIC BATH & BODY

USE FREQUENCIES DURING BATHING

639 Hz - Harmonizing Relationships
Benefits: Known to balance and harmonize relationships, this frequency fosters connection, love, and compassion.
Use in Bathing: Great for meditative baths focused on improving your relationship with yourself or others, enhancing feelings of connectedness.

174 Hz - Pain Relief
Benefits: This frequency is known for its ability to relieve physical and emotional pain, providing a grounding effect.
Use in Bathing: Ideal for a restorative bath, helping your body and mind recover from stress or injury, and alleviating physical discomfort.

741 Hz - Detox and Purification
Benefits: Associated with cleansing and removing toxins, this frequency helps in detoxifying the body and mind.
Use in Bathing: Perfect for a detox bath with salts or clays, as it enhances the purification process.

Theta Waves (4-8 Hz) - Deep Meditation
Benefits: Binaural beats in the theta range induce a deep meditative state, promoting creativity, intuition, and healing.
Use in Bathing: Best used for deep meditation and mental relaxation while soaking, helping you reach a trance-like state for healing and introspection.

Delta Waves (0.5-4 Hz) - Deep Sleep and Healing
Benefits: Binaural beats in this range are known for promoting deep, restorative sleep and healing.
Use in Bathing: Ideal for a night-time bath before bed, helping you relax deeply and prepare for a restful sleep.

Alpha Waves (8-14 Hz) - Stress Relief and Relaxation
Benefits: Alpha waves induce a relaxed yet alert state, reducing stress and promoting a sense of calm.
Use in Bathing: These beats are perfect for a calming bath aimed at unwinding after a stressful day.

852 Hz - Awakening Intuition
Benefits: This frequency is said to help raise your vibration and develop intuition and spiritual awareness.
Use in Bathing: Ideal for spiritual baths where you seek clarity and insight, helping you connect with your higher self and intuition.

BLUE SWAN COSMIC BATH & BODY

BATH SUPPLY CHECKLIST

(Fill in your preferred ingredients and
check them off before your bath session)

Supply Category Item Quantity/Details
Checked

Base Ingredients _________ _________ ☐
Carrier Oils _________ _________ ☐
Essential Oils _________ _________ ☐
Bath Salts _________ _________ ☐
Herbs/Flowers _________ _________ ☐
Milk/Clay _________ _________ ☐
Crystals _________ _________ ☐
Candles _________ _________ ☐
Music/Frequency _________ _________ ☐
Notes on Supplies:

BLUE SWAN COSMIC BATH & BODY

BATH MANIFESTATION SCRIPT

BATH MANIFESTATION SCRIPT
(Use this space to create your own bath manifestation
ritual. Fill in the blanks based on your intentions and goals.)

Date: _________
Time: _________
Moon Phase: _________

Affirmation for this bath:
"I manifest _________ as I immerse myself in this sacred
water."

Focus for this session:

Emotional Healing: _________
Physical Restoration: _________
Spiritual Connection: _________
Candles and Crystals used for manifestation:

Visualize the outcome:
"As the water cleanses my body, I release
_________ and attract _________. I feel light,
empowered, and deeply connected."

BLUE SWAN COSMIC BATH & BODY

BATH INVENTORY TRACKER
(Track your bath supplies and usage here for easy reordering and ensuring nothing is missed.)

Supply Date Purchased Amount Remaining Need to Reorder (Yes/No) Notes

Essential Oils ________ ________ ________ ______

Bath Salts ________ ________ ________ ______

Carrier Oils ________ ________ ________ ______

Herbs/Flowers ________ ________ ________ ______

Candles ________ ________ ________ ______

Inventory Notes:

____

____

____

BLUE SWAN COSMIC BATH & BODY

BATH JOURNAL PROMPTS

(Write your reflections after each bath to track progress
and enhance your self-care routine.)

How did I feel before the bath?

What ingredients and oils did I use?

What changes did I notice physically or emotionally?

How will I adjust my next bath based on this experience?

____

____

____

____

BLUE SWAN COSMIC BATH & BODY

The ideal bath temperature for relaxation, skin health, and overall well-being typically falls between 92°F to 101°F (33°C to 38°C). This temperature range is considered "warm" and offers a soothing, relaxing experience without being too hot, which can cause dehydration or stress to the skin.

Here's how different bath temperatures can impact your experience:

BLUE SWAN COSMIC BATH & BODY

BATH SUPPLY CHECKLIST

(Fill in your preferred ingredients and check them off before your bath session)

Supply Category Item Quantity/Details Checked

Base Ingredients __________ __________ ☐

Carrier Oils __________ __________ ☐

Essential Oils __________ __________ ☐

Bath Salts __________ __________ ☐

Herbs/Flowers __________ __________ ☐

Milk/Clay __________ __________ ☐

Crystals __________ __________ ☐

Candles __________ __________ ☐

Music/Frequency __________ __________ ☐

Notes on Supplies:

BLUE SWAN COSMIC BATH & BODY

BATH MANIFESTATION SCRIPT

BATH MANIFESTATION SCRIPT
(Use this space to create your own bath manifestation ritual. Fill in the blanks based on your intentions and goals.)

Date: _________
Time: _________
Moon Phase: _________

Affirmation for this bath:
"I manifest _________ as I immerse myself in this sacred water."

Focus for this session:

Emotional Healing: _________
Physical Restoration: _________
Spiritual Connection: _________
Candles and Crystals used for manifestation:

Visualize the outcome:
"As the water cleanses my body, I release _________ and attract _________. I feel light, empowered, and deeply connected."

BLUE SWAN COSMIC BATH & BODY

BATH INVENTORY TRACKER
(Track your bath supplies and usage here for easy reordering and ensuring nothing is missed.)

Supply Date Purchased Amount Remaining Need to Reorder (Yes/No) Notes

Essential Oils _________ _________ _________ _______

Bath Salts _________ _________ _________ _______

Carrier Oils _________ _________ _________ _______

Herbs/Flowers _________ _________ _________ _______

Candles _________ _________ _________ _______

Inventory Notes:

____

____

____

BLUE SWAN COSMIC BATH & BODY

BATH JOURNAL PROMPTS

(Write your reflections after each bath to track progress
and enhance your self-care routine.)

How did I feel before the bath?

What ingredients and oils did I use?

What changes did I notice physically or emotionally?

How will I adjust my next bath based on this experience?

____

____

____

____

BLUE SWAN COSMIC BATH & BODY

The ideal bath temperature for relaxation, skin health, and overall well-being typically falls between 92°F to 101°F (33°C to 38°C). This temperature range is considered "warm" and offers a soothing, relaxing experience without being too hot, which can cause dehydration or stress to the skin.

Here's how different bath temperatures can impact your experience:

BLUE SWAN COSMIC BATH & BODY
BATH SUPPLY CHECKLIST

(Fill in your preferred ingredients and
check them off before your bath session)

Supply Category Item Quantity/Details
Checked

Base Ingredients ________ ________ ☐
Carrier Oils ________ ________ ☐
Essential Oils ________ ________ ☐
Bath Salts ________ ________ ☐
Herbs/Flowers ________ ________ ☐
Milk/Clay ________ ________ ☐
Crystals ________ ________ ☐
Candles ________ ________ ☐
Music/Frequency ________ ________ ☐
Notes on Supplies:

BLUE SWAN COSMIC BATH & BODY

BATH MANIFESTATION SCRIPT

BATH MANIFESTATION SCRIPT
(Use this space to create your own bath manifestation ritual. Fill in the blanks based on your intentions and goals.)

Date: _________
Time: _________
Moon Phase: _________

Affirmation for this bath:
"I manifest _________ as I immerse myself in this sacred water."

Focus for this session:

Emotional Healing: _________
Physical Restoration: _________
Spiritual Connection: _________
Candles and Crystals used for manifestation:

Visualize the outcome:
"As the water cleanses my body, I release _________ and attract _________. I feel light, empowered, and deeply connected."

BLUE SWAN COSMIC BATH & BODY

BATH INVENTORY TRACKER
(Track your bath supplies and usage here for easy reordering and ensuring nothing is missed.)

Supply Date Purchased Amount Remaining Need to Reorder (Yes/No) Notes

Essential Oils ___________ ___________ ___________ ________

Bath Salts ___________ ___________ ___________ ________

Carrier Oils ___________ ___________ ___________ ________

Herbs/Flowers ___________ ___________ ___________ ________

Candles ___________ ___________ ___________ ________

Inventory Notes:

____

____

____

BLUE SWAN COSMIC BATH & BODY

BATH JOURNAL PROMPTS

(Write your reflections after each bath to track progress
and enhance your self-care routine.)

How did I feel before the bath?

What ingredients and oils did I use?

What changes did I notice physically or emotionally?

How will I adjust my next bath based on this experience?

____

____

____

____

BLUE SWAN COSMIC BATH & BODY

The ideal bath temperature for relaxation, skin health, and overall well-being typically falls between 92°F to 101°F (33°C to 38°C). This temperature range is considered "warm" and offers a soothing, relaxing experience without being too hot, which can cause dehydration or stress to the skin.

Here's how different bath temperatures can impact your experience:

BLUE SWAN COSMIC BATH & BODY

BATH SUPPLY CHECKLIST

(Fill in your preferred ingredients and
check them off before your bath session)

Supply Category Item Quantity/Details
Checked

Base Ingredients ________ ________ ☐
Carrier Oils ________ ________ ☐
Essential Oils ________ ________ ☐
Bath Salts ________ ________ ☐
Herbs/Flowers ________ ________ ☐
Milk/Clay ________ ________ ☐
Crystals ________ ________ ☐
Candles ________ ________ ☐
Music/Frequency ________ ________ ☐
Notes on Supplies:

BLUE SWAN COSMIC BATH & BODY

BATH MANIFESTATION SCRIPT

BATH MANIFESTATION SCRIPT
(Use this space to create your own bath manifestation ritual. Fill in the blanks based on your intentions and goals.)

Date: _________
Time: _________
Moon Phase: _________

Affirmation for this bath:
"I manifest _________ as I immerse myself in this sacred water."

Focus for this session:

Emotional Healing: _________
Physical Restoration: _________
Spiritual Connection: _________
Candles and Crystals used for manifestation:

Visualize the outcome:
"As the water cleanses my body, I release _________ and attract _________. I feel light, empowered, and deeply connected."

BLUE SWAN COSMIC BATH & BODY

BATH INVENTORY TRACKER
(Track your bath supplies and usage here for easy reordering and ensuring nothing is missed.)

Supply Date Purchased Amount Remaining Need to Reorder (Yes/No) Notes

Essential Oils __________ __________ __________ ______

Bath Salts __________ __________ __________ ______

Carrier Oils __________ __________ __________ ______

Herbs/Flowers __________ __________ __________ ______

Candles __________ __________ __________ ______

Inventory Notes:

____

____

____

BLUE SWAN COSMIC BATH & BODY

BATH JOURNAL PROMPTS

(Write your reflections after each bath to track progress
and enhance your self-care routine.)

How did I feel before the bath?

What ingredients and oils did I use?

What changes did I notice physically or emotionally?

How will I adjust my next bath based on this experience?

____

____

____

____

BLUE SWAN COSMIC BATH & BODY

The ideal bath temperature for relaxation, skin health, and overall well-being typically falls between 92°F to 101°F (33°C to 38°C). This temperature range is considered "warm" and offers a soothing, relaxing experience without being too hot, which can cause dehydration or stress to the skin.

Here's how different bath temperatures can impact your experience:

BLUE SWAN COSMIC BATH & BODY

BATH SUPPLY CHECKLIST

(Fill in your preferred ingredients and
check them off before your bath session)

Supply Category Item Quantity/Details
Checked

Base Ingredients ________ ________ ☐
Carrier Oils ________ ________ ☐
Essential Oils ________ ________ ☐
Bath Salts ________ ________ ☐
Herbs/Flowers ________ ________ ☐
Milk/Clay ________ ________ ☐
Crystals ________ ________ ☐
Candles ________ ________ ☐
Music/Frequency ________ ________ ☐
Notes on Supplies:

BLUE SWAN COSMIC BATH & BODY

BATH MANIFESTATION SCRIPT

BATH MANIFESTATION SCRIPT

(Use this space to create your own bath manifestation ritual. Fill in the blanks based on your intentions and goals.)

Date: _________
Time: _________
Moon Phase: _________

Affirmation for this bath:
"I manifest _________ as I immerse myself in this sacred water."

Focus for this session:

Emotional Healing: _________
Physical Restoration: _________
Spiritual Connection: _________
Candles and Crystals used for manifestation:

Visualize the outcome:
"As the water cleanses my body, I release _________ and attract _________. I feel light, empowered, and deeply connected."

BLUE SWAN COSMIC BATH & BODY

BATH INVENTORY TRACKER
(Track your bath supplies and usage here for easy reordering and ensuring nothing is missed.)

Supply Date Purchased Amount Remaining Need to Reorder (Yes/No) Notes

Essential Oils ___________ ___________ ___________ _______

Bath Salts ___________ ___________ ___________ _______

Carrier Oils ___________ ___________ ___________ _______

Herbs/Flowers ___________ ___________ ___________ _______

Candles ___________ ___________ ___________

Inventory Notes:

____

____

____

BLUE SWAN COSMIC BATH & BODY

BATH JOURNAL PROMPTS

(write your reflections after each bath to track progress
and enhance your self-care routine.)

How did I feel before the bath?

What ingredients and oils did I use?

What changes did I notice physically or emotionally?

How will I adjust my next bath based on this experience?

____

____

____

____

BLUE SWAN COSMIC BATH & BODY

The ideal bath temperature for relaxation, skin health, and overall well-being typically falls between 92°F to 101°F (33°C to 38°C). This temperature range is considered "warm" and offers a soothing, relaxing experience without being too hot, which can cause dehydration or stress to the skin.

Here's how different bath temperatures can impact your experience:

BLUE SWAN COSMIC BATH & BODY

BATH SUPPLY CHECKLIST

(Fill in your preferred ingredients and
check them off before your bath session)

Supply Category Item Quantity/Details
Checked

Base Ingredients ________ ________ ☐
Carrier Oils ________ ________ ☐
Essential Oils ________ ________ ☐
Bath Salts ________ ________ ☐
Herbs/Flowers ________ ________ ☐
Milk/Clay ________ ________ ☐
Crystals ________ ________ ☐
Candles ________ ________ ☐
Music/Frequency ________ ________ ☐

Notes on Supplies:

BLUE SWAN COSMIC BATH & BODY

BATH MANIFESTATION SCRIPT

BATH MANIFESTATION SCRIPT
(Use this space to create your own bath manifestation
ritual. Fill in the blanks based on your intentions and goals.)

Date: _________
Time: _________
Moon Phase: _________

Affirmation for this bath:
"I manifest _________ as I immerse myself in this sacred
water."

Focus for this session:

Emotional Healing: _________
Physical Restoration: _________
Spiritual Connection: _________
Candles and Crystals used for manifestation:

Visualize the outcome:
"As the water cleanses my body, I release
_________ and attract _________. I feel light,
empowered, and deeply connected."

BLUE SWAN COSMIC BATH & BODY

BATH INVENTORY TRACKER
(Track your bath supplies and usage here for easy reordering and ensuring nothing is missed.)

Supply Date Purchased Amount Remaining Need to Reorder (Yes/No) Notes

Essential Oils ___________ ___________ ___________ ___________

Bath Salts ___________ ___________ ___________ ___________

Carrier Oils ___________ ___________ ___________ ___________

Herbs/Flowers ___________ ___________ ___________ ___________

Candles ___________ ___________ ___________ ___________

Inventory Notes:

____

____

____

BLUE SWAN COSMIC BATH & BODY

BATH JOURNAL PROMPTS

(Write your reflections after each bath to track progress and enhance your self-care routine.)

How did I feel before the bath?

What ingredients and oils did I use?

What changes did I notice physically or emotionally?

How will I adjust my next bath based on this experience?

BLUE SWAN COSMIC BATH & BODY

The ideal bath temperature for relaxation, skin health, and overall well-being typically falls between 92°F to 101°F (33°C to 38°C). This temperature range is considered "warm" and offers a soothing, relaxing experience without being too hot, which can cause dehydration or stress to the skin.

Here's how different bath temperatures can impact your experience:

BLUE SWAN COSMIC BATH & BODY

BATH SUPPLY CHECKLIST

(Fill in your preferred ingredients and
check them off before your bath session)

Supply Category Item Quantity/Details
Checked

Base Ingredients ________ ________ ☐
Carrier Oils ________ ________ ☐
Essential Oils ________ ________ ☐
Bath Salts ________ ________ ☐
Herbs/Flowers ________ ________ ☐
Milk/Clay ________ ________ ☐
Crystals ________ ________ ☐
Candles ________ ________ ☐
Music/Frequency ________ ________ ☐
Notes on Supplies:

BLUE SWAN COSMIC BATH & BODY

BATH MANIFESTATION SCRIPT

BATH MANIFESTATION SCRIPT
(Use this space to create your own bath manifestation ritual. Fill in the blanks based on your intentions and goals.)

Date: _________
Time: _________
Moon Phase: _________

Affirmation for this bath:
"I manifest _________ as I immerse myself in this sacred water."

Focus for this session:

Emotional Healing: _________
Physical Restoration: _________
Spiritual Connection: _________
Candles and Crystals used for manifestation:

Visualize the outcome:
"As the water cleanses my body, I release _________ and attract _________. I feel light, empowered, and deeply connected."

BLUE SWAN COSMIC BATH & BODY

BATH INVENTORY TRACKER
(Track your bath supplies and usage here for easy reordering and ensuring nothing is missed.)

Supply Date Purchased Amount Remaining Need to Reorder (Yes/No) Notes

Essential Oils ________ ________ ________ ______

Bath Salts ________ ________ ________ ______

Carrier Oils ________ ________ ________ ______

Herbs/Flowers ________ ________ ________ ______

Candles ________ ________ ________ ______

Inventory Notes:

____

____

____

BLUE SWAN COSMIC BATH & BODY

BATH JOURNAL PROMPTS

(Write your reflections after each bath to track progress
and enhance your self-care routine.)

How did I feel before the bath?

What ingredients and oils did I use?

What changes did I notice physically or emotionally?

How will I adjust my next bath based on this experience?

____

____

____

____

BLUE SWAN COSMIC BATH & BODY

The ideal bath temperature for relaxation, skin health, and overall well-being typically falls between 92°F to 101°F (33°C to 38°C). This temperature range is considered "warm" and offers a soothing, relaxing experience without being too hot, which can cause dehydration or stress to the skin.

Here's how different bath temperatures can impact your experience:

BLUE SWAN COSMIC BATH & BODY

BATH SUPPLY CHECKLIST

(Fill in your preferred ingredients and check them off before your bath session)

Supply Category Item Quantity/Details Checked

Base Ingredients _________ _________ ☐
Carrier Oils _________ _________ ☐
Essential Oils _________ _________ ☐
Bath Salts _________ _________ ☐
Herbs/Flowers _________ _________ ☐
Milk/Clay _________ _________ ☐
Crystals _________ _________ ☐
Candles _________ _________ ☐
Music/Frequency _________ _________ ☐

Notes on Supplies:

BLUE SWAN COSMIC BATH & BODY

BATH MANIFESTATION SCRIPT

BATH MANIFESTATION SCRIPT
(Use this space to create your own bath manifestation ritual. Fill in the blanks based on your intentions and goals.)

Date: _________
Time: _________
Moon Phase: _________

Affirmation for this bath:
"I manifest _________ as I immerse myself in this sacred water."

Focus for this session:

Emotional Healing: _________
Physical Restoration: _________
Spiritual Connection: _________
Candles and Crystals used for manifestation:

Visualize the outcome:
"As the water cleanses my body, I release _________ and attract _________. I feel light, empowered, and deeply connected."

BLUE SWAN COSMIC BATH & BODY

BATH INVENTORY TRACKER
(Track your bath supplies and usage here for easy reordering and ensuring nothing is missed.)

Supply Date Purchased Amount Remaining Need to Reorder (Yes/No) Notes

Essential Oils _________ _________ _________ _______

Bath Salts _________ _________ _________ _______

Carrier Oils _________ _________ _________ _______

Herbs/Flowers _________ _________ _________ _______

Candles _________ _________ _________ _______

Inventory Notes:

____

____

____

BLUE SWAN COSMIC BATH & BODY

BATH JOURNAL PROMPTS

(Write your reflections after each bath to track progress
and enhance your self-care routine.)

How did I feel before the bath?

What ingredients and oils did I use?

What changes did I notice physically or emotionally?

How will I adjust my next bath based on this experience?

BLUE SWAN COSMIC BATH & BODY

The ideal bath temperature for relaxation, skin health, and overall well-being typically falls between 92°F to 101°F (33°C to 38°C). This temperature range is considered "warm" and offers a soothing, relaxing experience without being too hot, which can cause dehydration or stress to the skin.

Here's how different bath temperatures can impact your experience:

BLUE SWAN COSMIC BATH & BODY

BATH SUPPLY CHECKLIST

(Fill in your preferred ingredients and
check them off before your bath session)

Supply Category Item Quantity/Details
Checked

Base Ingredients ________ ________ ☐
Carrier Oils ________ ________ ☐
Essential Oils ________ ________ ☐
Bath Salts ________ ________ ☐
Herbs/Flowers ________ ________ ☐
Milk/Clay ________ ________ ☐
Crystals ________ ________ ☐
Candles ________ ________ ☐
Music/Frequency ________ ________ ☐

Notes on Supplies:

BLUE SWAN COSMIC BATH & BODY

BATH SUPPLY CHECKLIST

(Fill in your preferred ingredients and
check them off before your bath session)

Supply Category Item Quantity/Details
Checked

Base Ingredients _________ _________ ☐
Carrier Oils _________ _________ ☐
Essential Oils _________ _________ ☐
Bath Salts _________ _________ ☐
Herbs/Flowers _________ _________ ☐
Milk/Clay _________ _________ ☐
Crystals _________ _________ ☐
Candles _________ _________ ☐
Music/Frequency _________ _________ ☐
Notes on Supplies:

BLUE SWAN COSMIC BATH & BODY

BATH MANIFESTATION SCRIPT

BATH MANIFESTATION SCRIPT
(Use this space to create your own bath manifestation
ritual. Fill in the blanks based on your intentions and goals.)

Date: _________
Time: ________
Moon Phase: ________

Affirmation for this bath:
"I manifest ________ as I immerse myself in this sacred
water."

Focus for this session:

Emotional Healing: _________
Physical Restoration: ________
Spiritual Connection: ________
Candles and Crystals used for manifestation:

Visualize the outcome:
"As the water cleanses my body, I release
_________ and attract _________. I feel light,
empowered, and deeply connected."

BLUE SWAN COSMIC BATH & BODY

BATH INVENTORY TRACKER
(Track your bath supplies and usage here for easy reordering and ensuring nothing is missed.)

Supply Date Purchased Amount Remaining Need to Reorder (Yes/No) Notes

Essential Oils ________ ________ ________ ______

Bath Salts ________ ________ ________ ______

Carrier Oils ________ ________ ________ ______

Herbs/Flowers ________ ________ ________ ______

Candles ________ ________ ________ ______

Inventory Notes:

____

____

____

BLUE SWAN COSMIC BATH & BODY

BATH JOURNAL PROMPTS

(write your reflections after each bath to track progress
and enhance your self-care routine.)

How did I feel before the bath?

What ingredients and oils did I use?

What changes did I notice physically or emotionally?

How will I adjust my next bath based on this experience?

BLUE SWAN COSMIC BATH & BODY

BATH SUPPLY CHECKLIST

(Fill in your preferred ingredients and
check them off before your bath session)

Supply Category Item Quantity/Details
Checked

Base Ingredients _________ _________ ☐
Carrier Oils _________ _________ ☐
Essential Oils _________ _________ ☐
Bath Salts _________ _________ ☐
Herbs/Flowers _________ _________ ☐
Milk/Clay _________ _________ ☐
Crystals _________ _________ ☐
Candles _________ _________ ☐
Music/Frequency _________ _________ ☐
Notes on Supplies:

BLUE SWAN COSMIC BATH & BODY

BATH MANIFESTATION SCRIPT

BATH MANIFESTATION SCRIPT
(Use this space to create your own bath manifestation ritual. Fill in the blanks based on your intentions and goals.)

Date: _________
Time: ________
Moon Phase: ________

Affirmation for this bath:
"I manifest ________ as I immerse myself in this sacred water."

Focus for this session:

Emotional Healing: ________
Physical Restoration: ________
Spiritual Connection: ________
Candles and Crystals used for manifestation:

Visualize the outcome:
"As the water cleanses my body, I release ________ and attract ________. I feel light, empowered, and deeply connected."

BLUE SWAN COSMIC BATH & BODY

BATH INVENTORY TRACKER
(Track your bath supplies and usage here for easy reordering and ensuring nothing is missed.)

Supply Date Purchased Amount Remaining Need to Reorder (Yes/No) Notes

Essential Oils ________ ________ ________ ______

Bath Salts ________ ________ ________ ______

Carrier Oils ________ ________ ________ ______

Herbs/Flowers ________ ________ ________ ______

Candles ________ ________ ________ ______

Inventory Notes:

____

____

____

BLUE SWAN COSMIC BATH & BODY

BATH JOURNAL PROMPTS

(Write your reflections after each bath to track progress
and enhance your self-care routine.)

How did I feel before the bath?

What ingredients and oils did I use?

What changes did I notice physically or emotionally?

How will I adjust my next bath based on this experience?

____

____

____

____

BLUE SWAN COSMIC BATH & BODY

Conclusion

As we wrap up this cosmic journey, I want to remind you that self-care is not a luxury, it's a necessity. Every bath you take, every elixir you sip, and every ritual you perform is a powerful act of love—love for yourself and for the divine essence within you. May these rituals be a reminder that you are worthy of every ounce of joy, beauty, and peace that life has to offer. Now go forth, goddess, and continue to create your own magic!

BLUE SWAN COSMIC BATH & BODY

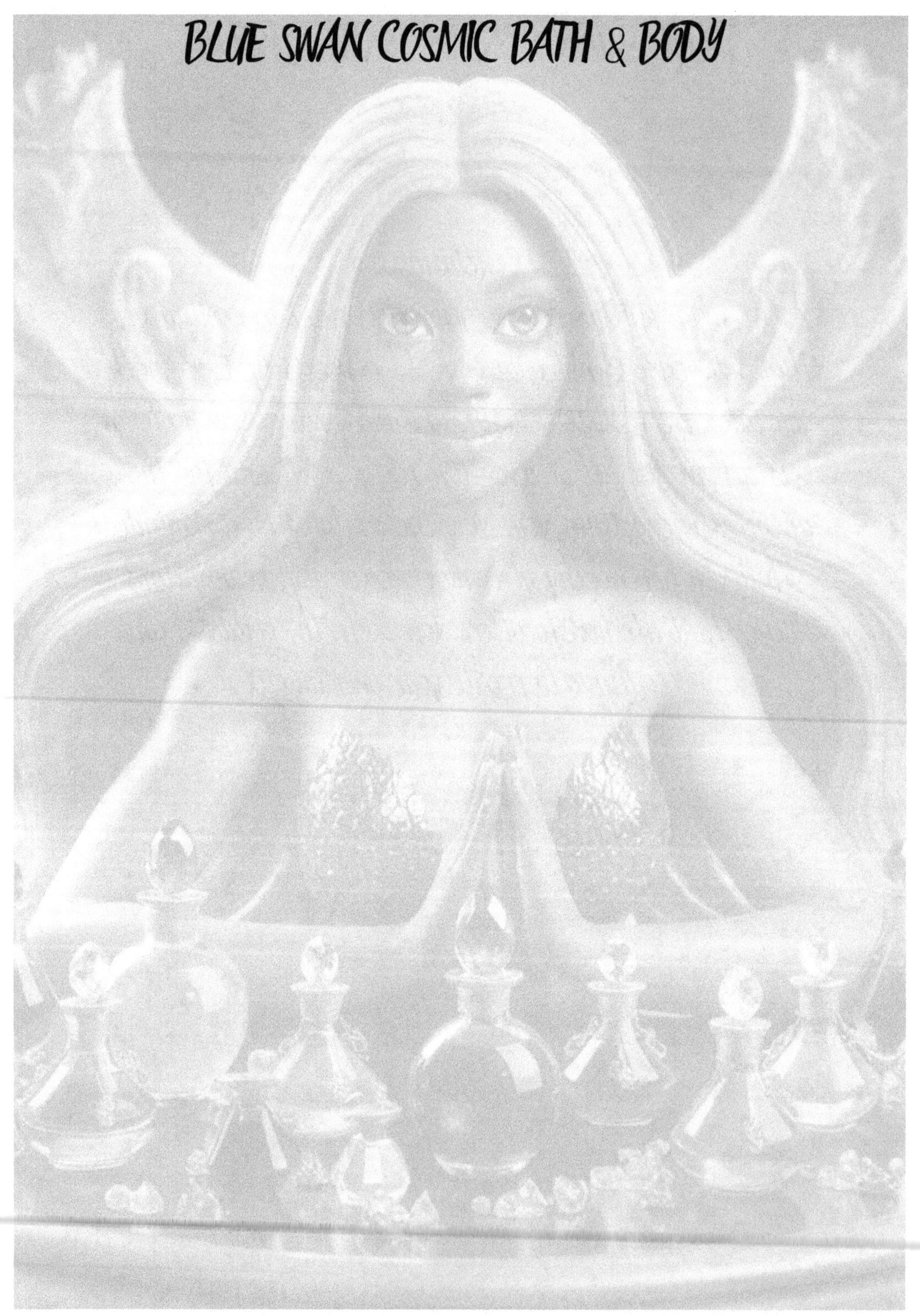